Healthy Habits for Fast Weight Loss

6 Easy Steps to Lose Weight and Get in Shape

Julie K. Geneva

Julie K. Geneva

Copyright © 2023 Julie K. Geneva
All rights reserved. No part of this book may be reproduced, stored in a retrieval system, or transmitted in any form or by any means, electronic, mechanical, photocopying, recording, or otherwise, without the prior written permission of the author, except for brief quotations in critical reviews or articles.

Julie K. Geneva

Contents

Introduction

Why Healthy Habits Are Essential for Weight Loss

It is not unusual to have feelings of being overwhelmed or disheartened when on the path to losing weight, since this is a journey that may be tough. Still, you might not know that doing healthy things on a regular basis can make all the difference in the world when it comes to losing weight quickly and for good. In fact, healthy habits are essential for losing weight. They can help you reach your goals without making you feel deprived, hungry, or overworked.

It is essential for one's general health and well-being to keep their weight within a healthy range. Not only may it lessen the likelihood of developing chronic illnesses like heart disease, diabetes, and some cancers, but it also has the potential to boost mental health and overall well-being.

Unfortunately, the number of overweight and obese people has risen dramatically in the last few years, causing more and more people to worry about their health.

There are a lot of individuals who have trouble losing weight, and as a result, they often look for fast solutions like fad diets, weight reduction drugs, and intense workout programs. On the other hand, these practices are often not sustainable and, in the long term, may be damaging to the health of the population as a whole. Instead, it's important to focus on developing healthy habits that can help you lose weight over time.

It is not necessary to starve yourself or keep track of your calorie intake in order to achieve a reduction in weight that is both healthy and long-term; rather, the secret is in developing good habits that are beneficial to your general health. *Habits* are defined as activities that are carried out on a regular basis, and they have the potential to have a significant influence on a person's physical, mental, and emotional well-being. If you do healthy things, you can speed up your metabolism, reduce inflammation, and get more energy. All of these things may make it easier for you to lose weight.

One of the most important reasons why healthy habits are essential for weight loss is that they help you create a lifestyle that supports your weight loss goals. Creating a lifestyle that supports your weight loss goals is one of the most important reasons why healthy habits are essential for weight loss.

There are a lot of individuals who make the mistake of treating weight reduction as a project that will only last for a limited period of time or as a diet that will only be temporary, but this strategy almost never results in success over the long run. Making adjustments to your lifestyle that are sustainable and that you can continue to keep up with over the long run is necessary if you want to see effects from your weight reduction effort that are long-lasting.

One other major reason why healthy habits are essential for weight reduction is that they assist you in developing a good connection between the foods you eat and the activities you do to keep your body in shape. If you focus, you could instead teach yourself to enjoy eating healthy foods, find new ways to exercise that excite you, and make it a priority in your life to take better care of yourself.

By making good habits, you will be less likely to give in to unhealthy ones, like following a diet that is too strict, binge eating, or exercising too much. You could instead teach yourself to enjoy eating healthy foods, find new ways to exercise that excite you, and make it a priority in your life to take better care of yourself.

In this book, we will discuss the significance of maintaining healthy behaviors in order to lose weight in a short amount of time. We'll look into the science and psychology that lie behind the creation of habits, and then we are going to examine a variety of healthy habits that may assist you in reaching your weight loss goals in a timely and efficient manner. We are going to talk about how eating, exercising, sleeping, managing stress, staying hydrated, and taking supplements all play a part in weight reduction, and then we are going to give you some practical advice on how you can incorporate these behaviors into your daily routine.

Chapter 1: Mindset Shift - How to Change Your Mindset for Successful Weight Loss

Before starting a plan to lose weight, it's important to have the right mindset. Changing your mind from having fixed beliefs to having growing beliefs could help you reach your weight loss goals. A fixed mindset is the exact opposite of a growth mindset. In a *fixed mindset,* you believe that your abilities and qualities are fixed and can't change. A fixed mindset can be contrasted with a growth mindset, which can be seen as the opposite of a growth mindset.

Having a *growth mindset* can help you deal with problems and setbacks and keep you motivated as you work to reach your goal of losing weight. To develop a growth mindset, it's important to keep an eye on your own progress and notice and celebrate even the smallest wins. Don't let failures stop you; instead, see them as chances to get better and take advantage of the lessons they teach you. You may approach your quest to lose weight with a good attitude and the idea that you can reach your goals if you have a growth mindset and adopt it before you start.

Chapter 2: Building Healthy Habits - The Science and Psychology Behind Habit Formation

Getting into good habits is important if you want to lose weight and keep it off for a long time because habits are the building blocks of a life. Habits are things we do regularly and automatically without putting in any effort or thinking about them. You will be able to create healthy habits that will support your efforts to lose weight if you have a grasp of the science and psychology that go into the creation of habits.

The "cue," the "routine," and the "reward" are the three essential elements that go into the establishment of a habit. The cue is the thing that starts the habit, the routine is the thing that is done, and the reward is the good thing that happens as a result of the routine that helps to keep it going. To get into the habit of being healthy, you should first determine the triggers that get your attention and then create a routine that helps you work toward your weight reduction objectives. The next step is to pick a reward that will both reinforce the behavior you want to see more of and help you stay motivated.

Chapter 3: Nutrition for Weight Loss - How to Eat for Optimal Weight Loss Results

A well-balanced diet is important for reaching your weight loss goals and is a big part of the process of getting rid of extra pounds. A balanced diet will contain many different types of foods that are high in nutrients, such as fruits, vegetables, whole grains, lean meats, and healthy fats. These meals not only give your body the nutrients it needs to work at its best, but they may also make you feel full for longer, making it less likely that you will eat more than you need.

Along with eating a well-balanced diet, controlling the size of your portions is an important part of losing weight. It is essential to keep track of the amount of food you consume on a daily basis in order to prevent excess weight gain, which may result from eating too much of anything, even nutritious meals. Keeping a food journal and eating in a mindful way can help you lose weight and develop a healthy relationship with food. Both of these strategies can help you create a healthy relationship with food.

Chapter 4: Exercise for Weight Loss - The Best Types of Exercises for Fast Results

Exercise is another important part of losing weight, and you need to make regular exercise a part of your daily routine if you want to reach your weight loss goals. Regular exercise can help you improve your overall health and well-being by helping you burn calories, build muscle, and improve your overall health. When it comes to shedding unwanted pounds, not all forms of exercise are made equal; in fact, there are certain forms of exercise that are more beneficial than others.

Resistance training, which is also sometimes called strength training or weightlifting, is one of the best ways to lose weight through physical activity. Taking part in resistance training may help you increase lean muscle mass, which in turn can help you burn more calories even when you're at rest. This means that your body burns more calories even when you're not working out than it would if you had less muscle mass. This is the case regardless of whether or not you are trying to lose weight.

HIIT, which stands for high-intensity interval training, is a good way to lose weight in addition to regular exercise. It has been shown that high-intensity interval training burns more calories than regular cardio activities like running or cycling. This is because high-intensity interval training is made up of short bursts of very intense activity followed by short rest periods.

Chapter 5: Sleep and Stress Management - The Importance of Rest and Recovery for Weight Loss

Stress management and getting enough sleep are two important parts of weight loss that are sometimes overlooked, even though they are important for a person's overall health and well-being. Since not getting enough sleep has been linked to more weight gain and a higher risk of becoming obese, it is a very important part of the process of losing weight. Try to get at least seven to eight hours of sleep every night, and make sure you have excellent sleep hygiene by doing things like not looking at devices in the hours leading up to bedtime and developing a pattern that helps you wind down before going to sleep.

Since chronic stress can cause people to eat too much, which can make them gain weight, stress can also make it hard to lose weight. By doing things like yoga, meditation, and deep breathing to deal with stress, you can improve your health and well-being and make it easier to stick to your weight loss goals.

Chapter 6: Hydration - Why Water Is Key to Losing Weight and Maintaining Good Health

Maintaining a healthy level of hydration all day is important for both losing weight and staying healthy in general. It is also needed for a wide range of biological processes, such as digestion, metabolism, and the control of body temperature, to work well. Drinking water causes you to experience satiety, which makes it less likely that you will overindulge in food. It is also needed for a wide range of biological processes, such as digestion, metabolism, and the control of body temperature, to work well.

Try to consume at least 8–10 glasses of water every day, and think about adding additional hydrating liquids like herbal tea or coconut water to your regular regimen. Moreover, be sure to keep an eye on how much sugary beverages you consume, such as soda and sports drinks, since drinking too much of these has been linked to an increase in body fat as well as a number of other health problems.

Chapter 7: Superfoods - Natural Ways to Boost Your Metabolism and Promote Weight Loss

Even though they aren't meant to replace a healthy diet and regular exercise, and "superfoods" can be a helpful part of a plan to lose weight if they are used along with those two key parts. Using certain superfoods can speed up the metabolism, reduce inflammation, and improve overall health and well-being.

Some dietary supplements and superfoods, like green tea extract, omega-3 fatty acids, and turmeric, may help you lose weight. Talk to a qualified medical professional about all of your options before taking any kind of dietary supplement. This is because some supplements might interfere with the effects of certain drugs or cause unpleasant side effects.

Chapter 8: Intermittent Fasting - The Benefits of Fasting and How to Incorporate It into Your Life

Intermittent fasting is the practice of alternating times when you don't eat with times when you do. It is a popular way to get rid of extra body fat. It has been found to have many health benefits, such as helping people lose weight, making insulin work better, and reducing inflammation.

Intermittent fasting is one method that may be used to achieve these health benefits.

There are several variations of the fasting method known as intermittent fasting. Some of these variations include eating at certain times, fasting every other day, and fasting for short periods of time. Before you start any kind of fasting plan, you should talk to a doctor and choose an intermittent fasting protocol that fits your lifestyle and your health needs.

Chapter 9: Sustainable Weight Loss - How to Maintain Your Results and Live a Healthy Lifestyle

Getting rapid weight reduction is a step in the right direction, but keeping the results off for the long term and leading a healthy lifestyle are two very different challenges. In this part of the article, we are going to talk about how important it is to lose weight in a way that is sustainable, and then we are going to share some advice on how to keep the results you have achieved over time. In addition to this, we will discuss the idea of leading a healthy lifestyle and discuss ways in which you may make changes in your behavior that are lasting and contribute to your efforts to lose weight and improve your general health.

Chapter 10: Common Obstacles and How to Overcome Them: Tips for Sticking to Your Weight Loss Goals

The process of losing weight is seldom a straight line, and there are a lot of frequent roadblocks that might derail your progress at any point. In this part of the article, we'll talk about some of the most common problems that people have when trying to lose weight and give suggestions for how to deal with them. We are going to cover everything, from how to handle cravings and temptation to how to behave in social settings and while traveling.

In a nutshell, in order to lose weight rapidly and healthily, one has to adopt. You can reach your weight loss goals and improve your overall health if you commit to doing the things listed above every day and make them a part of your routine. a complete plan that includes good habits, intermittent fasting, staying healthy, and getting over frequent obstacles.

You can reach your weight loss goals and improve your overall health if you commit to doing the things listed above every day and make them a part of your routine. In the last chapter of this book, we will go over specific activities that may be taken in order to put these tactics into action and get the kind of results that you are looking for. Let's dive in!

Chapter 1

Mindset Shift - How to Change Your Mindset for Successful Weight Loss

The way a person thinks, feels, and sees themselves in terms of their ability to lose weight and keep a healthy lifestyle is called their "weight loss mindset." It is made up of many different mental and emotional parts, such as motivation, self-efficacy, optimism, and resilience, among many others. One of the most important parts of a positive mindset for losing weight is having a growth mindset.

A growth mindset is one in which a person feels that they can change and improve their health by working hard, dedicating themselves, and being ready to learn and adapt to new situations. This way of thinking is important if you want to overcome challenges, keep yourself motivated, lose weight, and get healthier over the long term.

Importance of Mindset in Weight Loss

It is impossible to say enough about how important it is to have the right mindset when trying to lose weight. In fact, it is often thought to be the most important part of reducing body fat over the long term. The way a person thinks about the world impacts their ideas, attitudes, and behaviors, which in turn determine the choices they make and the results they get in life.

When it comes to getting rid of excess weight, having a mentality that is set in its ways might be counterproductive. People with a fixed mentality think that their skills and traits are permanent and can't be changed by their surroundings. They might have the mistaken belief that their weight is fixed and that there is nothing they can do about it, which would result in emotions of helplessness, despair, and discouragement. This way of thinking could stop people from taking action, making the changes they need to make, and staying committed to their weight loss goals.

On the other hand, a growth mindset is based on the idea that skills and traits can be developed and improved through hard work and commitment. This is different from having a "fixed mentality," which is the idea that a person's talents and qualities are set. People with a growth mindset are more likely to be tough, flexible, and willing to learn new ideas and strategies. Because of how they think, they are more likely to see problems and failures as opportunities for growth and progress rather than as roadblocks.

Research has shown that people with a growth mentality are more likely to reach their weight loss goals than those with a fixed perspective. They are better able to keep going when things get hard, more likely to ask for help and support, and more eager to try new things. People may be helped to overcome self-doubt, fear of failure, and other psychological obstacles that may keep them from making good changes in their lives by adopting a growth mindset. This attitude emphasizes learning and personal development rather than fixed beliefs about one's abilities.

Changing one's mentality in order to lose weight is something that can be done, but it is not always simple to do. Keeping track of when you say negative things to yourself that don't help and finding ways to replace them with more helpful positive affirmations is a good practice. For instance, rather than stating anything along the lines of "I'll never be able to lose weight," you may say something along the lines of "I am capable of bringing about significant changes in my lifestyle." One way to do this is to set goals that can be reached and then treat yourself when you reach even the smallest of those goals. This could make it easier to have a growth-oriented mindset and get things moving.

A person's attitude about losing weight can be changed by getting help and advice from friends, family, or a health professional. This can be an effective strategy to adjust one's perspective. Participating in a weight loss group, working with a qualified nutritionist, or working out on your own with a personal trainer are all options that may provide accountability, inspiration, and a sense of being a respected and important part of the community.

It can't be stressed enough how important it is to keep a positive mental attitude while trying to lose weight. People who have a growth mindset are better able to overcome mental obstacles, keep going when things get hard, and eventually reach their weight loss goals. Anyone is capable of making beneficial changes in their lives and living a life that is healthier and more meaningful with the correct frame of mind.

How to Cultivate a Growth Mindset for Successful Weight Loss

To cultivate a growth mindset for successful weight loss, it's essential to change your perspective and approach to the journey. Here are some ways to do this:

- *Focus on Progress, Not Perfection:* Having a growth mindset is important for losing weight, and one of the most important things you can do to develop this mindset is to focus on making progress instead of trying to be perfect. It requires changing your perspective from one that takes an all-or-nothing approach to one that takes a more optimistic and encouraging stance on the road you are on to lose weight. Put your attention on how far you've come toward achieving your weight reduction objectives rather than fixating on the number that appears on the scale or any particular number at all.

Celebrating your accomplishments, no matter how minor, is a great way to keep your mind on the big picture of growth. For example, if you've been working out regularly for the last week, you should be proud of yourself and celebrate. Instead, if you have been picking better options when it comes to eating, give yourself credit for the hard work and effort that you have put in. Even though each of these things may not seem important on its own, they may add up over time and make it easier for you to keep a positive attitude and stay motivated as you work toward your goal of losing weight.

Keeping tabs on your own advancement is another method for keeping your attention on your goals. Monitoring your advancement might assist you in seeing how far you've come and serve as a source of motivation to keep pushing forward with your goals. You can keep track of your progress by writing down what you eat, taking pictures of yourself, or figuring out how much body fat you have. This way, you'll be able to see your progress, even if the scale doesn't show it.

It is essential to keep in mind that the process of shedding extra pounds is not a straight line, and that you may expect to experience some obstacles along the way. It is essential, in the face of obstacles, to recognize them for what they are and then go on with the endeavor. Instead of letting failures get you down, use them to learn new things and get better at what you already know. Consider what could have led to the setback, as well as what you might do better the next time around. You may develop a growth mentality and keep making strides toward the achievement of your weight reduction objectives if you do this.

Therefore, if you want to lose weight effectively, you need to develop a "growth mindset." One of the most important parts of this mindset is to focus on making progress instead of trying to be perfect. You can keep a good attitude and stay motivated while losing weight if you celebrate even the smallest wins, keep careful track of your progress, and remember what you've learned from your failures.

- *Embrace Challenges:* Any attempt to lose weight is bound to run into problems and stumbling blocks along the way. It's possible that you'll reach a point in your weight loss journey when you reach a plateau and stop losing weight. You might also find it hard to fight the urge to eat too many unhealthy foods or to keep up with your workout routine. It's important to accept these problems and see them as chances to get better, not as failures, because that's how you'll get the most out of them.

You can go from feeling like you can't do anything to feeling like you can by just accepting problems and seeing them as part of your journey. When you face problems, you have the chance to grow as a person by learning from them and getting better at what you do. If you're trying to lose weight and you reach a point where you seem to be stuck, for instance, you may look at this as an opportunity to reevaluate your food and exercise regimen and make any necessary modifications so that you can keep making progress.

Also, rising to the challenge and making the best of a bad situation may help build mental strength and resilience. When you put yourself in tough situations and come out on top, you feel more confident in your ability to handle tough situations in the future. This might make it easier for you to stay motivated and committed to your weight loss goals, even if you have a few setbacks along the way.

Try reframing the way you think about obstacles so that you can more easily accept them. Consider the problems you face as opportunities to learn and grow, not as things that will stop you from moving forward. Focus on the process of overcoming the obstacle instead of just the result. If you do this, you will be able to handle problems better because you will have a more positive view of them.

- *Learn from Setbacks:* Any individual who attempts to lose weight will inevitably encounter obstacles along the way. In spite of your best efforts, there will likely be moments when you do not achieve the progress you had hoped for or when you come across unanticipated hurdles that slow down your development. On the other hand, it is essential to understand that failures are not the same thing as setbacks, which are chances to learn and advance.

It is quite easy to feel disheartened and give up on your objectives of losing weight when you have failures along the way. You can, however, turn a bad experience into a chance to learn if you change your perspective and see problems as chances to move forward. This will change the negative experience into a good one. The first thing that must be done is an analysis to determine what went wrong and why. This requires you to take an objective look at your routines, actions, and thinking, and to pinpoint the areas in which you can benefit from making some changes.

Secondly, focus your attention on the things that you can alter for the time being and go ahead. Think about the several approaches you may use to get beyond the obstacle and keep moving forward with your plans despite the setback you've experienced. This might include experimenting with a new workout program, making changes to your nutrition, or looking for help from friends or a trained expert.

When you make a mistake, you shouldn't criticize or berate yourself in any way, because that will only make things worse. Instead, you should try to deal with the situation with a growth mindset and a sense of self-compassion. Be conscious of the fact that experiencing difficulties along the way to one's goal weight reduction is something that happens to everyone and is a natural and expected part of the process. You will be able to keep making progress toward your weight loss goals and eventually reach long-term success if you are willing to learn from your mistakes and see them as opportunities to develop further as a person.

- *Develop a Positive Self-Image*: One of the most important things to do in order to successfully lose weight and develop a growth mindset is to create a positive image of yourself. The way in which you think about yourself has a tremendous impact on both your frame of mind and your level of motivation. If you have a poor perception of yourself, it may be easy to feel dejected and uninspired, both of which can sabotage your efforts to lose weight, so it's essential that you put some effort into improving this part of your life. On the other side, if you have a healthy, positive image of yourself, it will be easier for you to feel confident and driven, which will make it simpler to achieve your objectives.

In order to cultivate a healthy sense of self-image, you should begin by focusing your attention on the aspects of your physical appearance that you like and admire. Instead of picking holes in your character and pointing out your shortcomings, you should concentrate on your virtues and the strides you've achieved. This helps you go from having a negative mindset to having a positive one, and it may also help you generate confidence and motivation inside yourself.

You could also work on improving how you take care of yourself to build a good image of yourself. Self-care is really important. Taking better care of yourself on all fronts—physically, emotionally, and mentally—can boost your self-esteem and contribute to an overall improvement in your health and well-being. Getting enough sleep, eating a healthy, well-balanced diet, exercising regularly, practicing mindfulness and meditation, and doing all of these things on a regular basis are all examples of self-care activities that you could do.

Also, spend time with people who are positive and helpful and who will inspire and motivate you. It is much simpler to have a good frame of mind and continue to make progress toward your weight reduction objectives when you have a solid network of people to lean on for assistance.

If you have a positive view of yourself, you can develop a growth mindset, which will help you deal with problems and failures, stay motivated, and lose weight in the short- and long-term.

Having a growth mindset is important for successfully losing weight, and self-compassion is one of the most important parts of this mindset. Negative self-talk can make it hard to stay motivated and grow, and many people are often their own harshest critics. When things don't go according to plan on a quest to lose weight, it may be easy to slip into a loop of self-blame, self-doubt, and self-criticism. This can be very detrimental.

On the other hand, if you treat yourself with care, concern, and understanding, it will be easier for you to recover from setbacks and continue making progress. Self-compassion means understanding that mistakes are a normal and unavoidable part of life and that your mistakes do not define who you are as a person.

- *Practice Self-Compassion:* The first step to developing self-compassion is to become aware of any critical or negative conversations you may be having with yourself. As soon as you become aware of a negative thought, you should replace it with something positive and friendly. For instance, rather than using "for example," you may use "for." " Instead of saying, "I can't believe I did that to myself by eating that," try saying, "It's alright for that awful day to occur. I'm going to choose things that will be better for me moving forward.

Self-care activities are ones that make you feel good and nourish both your physical and emotional well-being. Doing these activities may be another useful step toward improving your overall health. They might include things like meditating, doing yoga, keeping a journal, or spending time in nature. Taking care of oneself in this manner will help you create a healthy self-image and keep motivation high while you are on your quest to lose weight.

- *Set Realistic Goals:* One of the most important things to do if you want to lose weight and develop a growth mindset is to set goals that are both reasonable and doable. Setting goals that are impossible to achieve is stressful, and it's easy to lose motivation when you don't see results as soon as you anticipated. Because of this, it is important to set goals that are both reasonable and doable.

  To be realistic, goals must be clear, measurable, and have a deadline. If you have clear goals that are specific to what you want to achieve, you might be able to focus your efforts in the right direction. Your ability to assess your development and evaluate how far you've come may be gauged by setting objectives that can be measured. Time-bound goals give you a deadline to which you can direct your efforts and help you stay accountable.

For instance, rather than making a goal as general as "reduce weight," make a goal as precise as "drop ten pounds in ten weeks by following a healthy food plan and exercising three times a week." This will help you stay motivated and on track. Since this objective is explicit, quantifiable, and time-bound, it will be much simpler to monitor progress and maintain a sense of motivation.

It is also essential to work toward objectives that can really be accomplished. Even though it's nice to have large objectives, it's vital to break them down into smaller goals that are more attainable. This makes it easier for you to notice improvement and maintain your motivation as you go forward. For instance, if your long-term objective is to lose fifty pounds, you should break this goal down into more manageable chunks, such as shedding five pounds in the first month or achieving a smaller clothing size in three months.

It's important to have a growth mindset if you want to lose weight, and one of the best ways to do that is to set goals that are both easy and hard to reach. Specific, measurable, and time-bound goals help you stay focused and motivated. Goals that are both attainable and challenging help you show progress and stay inspired along the way.

- *Surround Yourself with Support:* In order to successfully lose weight and cultivate a growth mentality, one of the most important things you can do is surround yourself with people who will encourage you. People in your life who are positive about your efforts to lose weight and give you support and encouragement can do a lot for your motivation, self-confidence, and general well-being.

Including one's family and friends in one's efforts to lose weight is one approach to increasing the amount of support one has around them. Talk to them about your plans, and explain how they can help you achieve your objectives. This might be as easy as asking them to check in on your progress or workout with you. Having a training partner can make physical activity more fun and help you stay on track with your fitness routine.

Joining a support group for people who are trying to lose weight is another way to surround yourself with people who can provide encouragement and advice. People who attend these kinds of events may feel like they are part of a community and have a sense of responsibility, in addition to getting useful information and tools. You may find support groups in person or online, and they can vary from organized programs to ad hoc get-togethers of people who are going through something similar.

It is essential that you acknowledge the possibility that some of the people in your life may not encourage you on your path to lose weight. There is a chance that some individuals may undermine your efforts or even try to discourage you. In situations like these, the appropriate response is

It's important to set limits and limit your relationships with these people while also getting support from people who lift you up and encourage you.

It is essential, when necessary, to look for professional help as well as lean on friends and family for assistance. Your doctor, a registered dietitian, or a certified personal trainer may be able to give you helpful advice and in-depth knowledge that can help you reach your weight loss goals. In addition, they will help you make a plan that fits your needs and set goals that can be reached.

If you want to successfully lose weight and establish a development mentality, one of the most important things you can do is surround yourself with supportive people. It has the potential to keep you motivated, accountable, and confident in your capacity to do whatever it is that you set out to do. Get the assistance you need to help you achieve success over the long term, whether it be from family and friends, support groups, or the supervision of a professional.

If you have a growth mindset, you may be more positive and hopeful about your efforts to lose weight. This will help you have a positive and hopeful outlook on your journey to lose weight. This makes it easier for you to maintain your motivation, get through obstacles, and accomplish your objectives in a manner that is both healthy and long-term.

Chapter 2

Building Healthy Habits: The Science and Psychology Behind Habit Formation

One of the most important things that helps people lose weight is getting into and keeping healthy habits. A behavior pattern can be called a habit if it is formed through repetition and reinforcement. They play a big role in how well our efforts to keep or improve our health work. You can learn how to build and keep healthy habits that help you reach your weight loss goals if you first learn about the science and psychology behind how habits are formed.

The Habit Loop

The habit loop is a way of thinking about how habits are formed and kept. It looks simple, but it actually gives a full explanation of how habits are formed and kept. It lays out a plan for how we can set up and change habits to move toward our goals and gives us a road map for how to do this. Finding the habit's "trigger," "routine," and "reward" is the first thing you need to do in order to use the habit loop effectively in order to modify a habit. As soon as you have a firm grasp on these aspects, you will be able to start making adjustments to the procedure while maintaining the same cue and reward.

The cue, also known as the trigger or the prompt, is what gets the habit started. It might be a particular time of day, a certain place, a particular feeling, or an action by someone else. For some people, a sign that it's time to check their social media accounts is the onset of boredom, while for others, it's the appearance of a notification on their phone.

The actual action or habit that is done when the cue is given is the "routine." It is what the cue "triggers." This might be a physical movement, such as reaching for a cigarette, or it can be a mental activity, such as concentrating on bad ideas.

The habit's reward is any good thing that happens or feeling that you get from doing the behavior. It could be a physical feeling, like a rush of dopamine after eating sweets, or an emotional one, like relief from stress or worry. Both of these are examples.

In order to break a habit, you must first recognize the "cue" that triggers it, as well as the "reward" that the habit provides, and then choose an alternative behavior that is more beneficial but still provides the same result. For example, if you always eat ice cream when you feel anxious, the feeling of anxiety could be the cue, eating ice cream could be the routine, and a short relief from the anxiety could be the reward. You can still get the reward of stress relief even if you consume unhealthy foods if you replace the routine of eating ice cream with a healthier routine, such as going for a walk or doing a meditation exercise, for example. This will allow you to avoid the negative effects of consuming unhealthy foods while still getting the reward of stress relief.

It is essential to keep in mind that the establishment of habits requires both time and repeated practice. The length of time it takes to form a new routine may range anywhere from 21 to 66 days, depending on the nature of the habit, the individual's level of desire, and the degree to which they are consistent in their efforts. On the other hand, if you are able to comprehend and make use of the habit loop, you will be able to establish long-lasting, healthy habits that will support your efforts to lose weight.

The Role of Consistency and Repetition

Since habits are formed through a process of reinforcement, consistency and repetition are two things that are very important for making habits. When we do the same thing over and over again and then get a good result or reward, our brains start to connect that behavior with the good result or reward. Because of this link, we are more likely to repeat the behavior in question again in the future.

For instance, if you want to make a routine out of going for a run first thing in the morning, it's important to keep doing it on a regular basis, even for a few minutes daily. It's likely that you'll keep going for runs because, over time, you'll start to associate the good feeling of being energized and refreshed after a run with the habit of going for a run. This will make it more likely that you will continue to do it in the future.

Repetition is also important because it helps strengthen the neural connections in our brains that are linked to the habit. This is one of the reasons why habits are so crucial to our lives. When we do the same thing over and over again, the brain connections get stronger. This makes the habit more automatic and easier to do without having to think about it.

To get into a new routine, you must act in a reliable way and do the activity often. It is also vital to begin the habit at a manageable level of difficulty and to progressively raise both the difficulty and the length of the habit over time. If you want to develop the routine of eating more vegetables, for instance, you might begin by including one serving of vegetables in each of your meals on a daily basis, and then gradually increase the quantity over the course of some time.

Keeping track of your progress might not only help you stay consistent, but it might also keep you motivated. Keeping a journal or using an app that tracks habits can help you see how well you're doing over time and give you a sense of accomplishment, which can be motivating and help you stick with the habit even more. Keeping a journal or using an app can also help you monitor your progress over time.

In general, to make a habit, you need to be consistent and do it over and over again. If you are patient, don't give up, and keep track of your progress, you can develop healthy habits that will become second nature to you. These habits will assist you in achieving your weight reduction objectives.

The Power of Belief and Self-Efficacy

Belief and self-efficacy are two important psychological characteristics that may have a significant influence on our capacity to create and keep habits. Self-efficacy is how much a person thinks he or she is able to do a certain job or reach a certain goal. Self-efficacy is an important factor that tells us if we can change our behavior and make new habits. This factor comes into play specifically in the context of habit formation.

If we lack self-efficacy and don't feel that we can effectively create a new habit, we are less likely to even try to alter our behavior. If we do seek to modify our behavior, we are more likely to be successful. On the other side, if we have a strong sense of self-efficacy and believe in our capacity to change, we will have a better chance of being successful in developing new habits and making good changes in our lives.

Two good ways to boost one's sense of self-efficacy are to start with tasks that are easy to do and to focus on reaching one's goals. This lets us have success early on, which gives us confidence in our ability to adapt to new situations. For instance, if you want to begin exercising on a more consistent basis, you can start by committing to only ten minutes of exercise every day. As you get more comfortable with how often you can work out, you can gradually increase both the length and intensity of your workouts.

In addition to this, it is essential to take time along the way to celebrate your accomplishments and give yourself credit for the progress you have made. This could help you feel more confident in yourself and keep you motivated to keep making big changes in your life. You might give yourself a prize if you stick to your healthy eating plan for a week or if you exercise every day for a week.

When it comes to the process of developing good habits, the importance of having strong beliefs and a strong sense of one's own ability cannot be stressed enough. You may be more likely to succeed at picking up new, healthy habits if you have faith in your ability to change and enjoy your small wins along the way. This will help you feel more motivated to stick with your plan.

Chapter 3

Nutrition for Weight Loss: How to Eat for Optimal Weight Loss Results

To get the best results while trying to lose weight, you need to pay attention to having a diet that is both healthy and well-balanced. This should be in line with the goals you have set for yourself. Have the following fundamentals in mind as you go forward:

Caloric deficit

Putting your body into a state of caloric deficit is one of the most important steps in the process of losing weight because it forces your body to utilize fat reserves as a source of energy. When you eat less than your body needs to stay at the same weight, your body will use fat stores for energy. This will cause you to lose weight. There are two primary approaches that may be taken in order to generate a caloric deficit. Some of these ways are to eat less and move more.

- *Reducing Calorie Intake:* Taking in fewer calories than your body requires is one of the most important steps you can take to begin the process of building a calorie deficit in your diet. Using a calorie calculator that takes into consideration your age, gender, height, weight, and activity level is the most accurate way to estimate the number of calories you need to consume on a daily basis. Once you know how many calories you need every day, you can create a caloric deficit by cutting your daily calorie intake by between 500 and 1000 calories. This may be accomplished by eating smaller quantities, selecting selections that are lower in calories, and refraining from consuming foods and drinks that are high in calories.

- *Increasing Physical Activity:* Raising the Amount You Spend Doing Physical Activity Increasing the amount of time you spend doing physical exercise is another method for producing a calorie deficit. When you do physical activities, your body will burn calories, which will help create a calorie deficit. The number of calories burned during exercise is directly related to both the type of activity and how hard it is done. It is crucial to participate in activities that you love and that challenge you if you want to get the most out of the calories that you burn. Activities such as walking, jogging, swimming, cycling, and weightlifting may fall into this category. In addition, increasing the amount of physical activity that you do on a daily basis, such as using the stairs rather than the elevator or walking rather than driving, may also help to raise the number of calories that you burn.

- *Combining Strategies:* Combining the two strategies of reducing calorie intake and increasing physical activity may be a good way to create a bigger caloric deficit and reach weight loss goals faster. It is vital to keep in mind that a modest calorie deficit of between 500 and 1000 calories per day is typically regarded as safe and sustainable, but bigger deficits may not be sustainable or healthy in the long term..

Macronutrient balance

"Macronutrient balance" means that your diet has the right amount of carbs, proteins, and fats to help you reach the level of body fat you want. It is important to get the right amount of each macronutrient if you want to be as healthy as possible and lose weight the way you want to. This is because each macronutrient plays an important function in the body.

There are two different kinds of carbohydrates: simple and complicated. Carbohydrates are the major source of energy for your body, and they may be either simple or complex. While simple carbs, such as those found in refined sugars and processed meals, are a fast way to get a burst of energy, they also tend to be rich in calories and may induce increases in blood sugar if consumed in large quantities. Complex carbs, on the other hand, may be found in whole grains, fruits, and vegetables. These types of carbohydrates give sustained energy as well as critical nutrients.

High-protein foods include meat, fish, eggs, and beans. Protein is necessary for the growth and repair of tissues in your body, and it can be found in all of these dietary sources. Eating enough protein is important if you want to keep from losing muscle mass as you lose weight. Protein may also make you feel fuller for a longer period of time, which can help you eat less often throughout the day.

Fat is another important macronutrient. They not only help the body make energy, but they also help the body absorb vitamins and play a role in controlling hormones. Nevertheless, not all fats are created equal, and it is crucial to pick healthy fats such as those found in nuts, seeds, and fatty fish while limiting saturated and trans fats found in fried meals and processed snacks. Healthy fats may be found in foods such as nuts, seeds, and fatty fish.

Carbohydrates make up about 10–35% of the calories in a balanced diet, while protein makes up about 10–35% of the calories, and fat makes up about 20–35% of the calories in a balanced diet. But the exact ratios can be different for each person, depending on their needs and food preferences. You must talk to a qualified medical professional or a certified dietitian about your weight loss goals in order to figure out the right ratio of macronutrients to reach those goals.

Whole foods

Whole foods are foods that haven't been processed or refined much, if at all. They still have all the vitamins, minerals, and fiber that nature gave them. Whole foods are also known as "natural foods." These types of foods are highly recommended for a healthy diet, and if you want to lose body fat, you should put more emphasis on eating more of them. Because they are typically lower in calories, high in fiber and other essential nutrients, and can help you feel full and satisfied for longer, whole foods are beneficial for weight loss. This is because they keep you from feeling hungry between meals, which makes it less likely that you will eat too much.

Fruits, vegetables, legumes, nuts, seeds, and lean proteins like chicken, fish, and tofu are all examples of whole foods. Whole grains, nuts, and seeds are all examples of whole grains. These foods are a great source of vitamins, minerals, antioxidants, and fiber, all of which are important for keeping your health in good shape and may help you lose weight.

On the other side, processed foods often have a large amount of added sugars, harmful fats, and salt, but they typically contain a low amount of nutrients. When one's goal is to reduce their overall body fat percentage, it is important to steer clear of or consume as little of these categories of foods as possible. Snacks that come in packages, beverages with a lot of added sugar, and fast meals are all examples of processed foods.

When trying to eat more whole foods, you should focus on eating more fruits and vegetables, whole grains, and lean proteins. You may also replace processed snacks with choices such as fresh fruit, raw vegetables with hummus, or roasted almonds rather than eating those processed snacks. Making a few simple adjustments to your eating routine over the course of some time may have a significant impact on your general health as well as the amount of weight you are able to lose.

Portion control

Controlling your portion sizes is a key part of successfully managing your weight because it helps you keep track of how many calories you eat every day. If you eat a lot, it can be easy to overeat, which can make it hard to lose weight. So, it's important to pay attention to the sizes of the portions you eat and use measuring tools, like a food scale, to help you stay on track with your weight loss goals.

Using the "plate technique" as a means of controlling the amount of food you put on each plate is a simple and effective strategy. Half of your plate should be non-starchy vegetables like leafy greens, broccoli, or carrots. The other half should be lean protein like chicken, fish, or tofu. The last quarter of your plate should be whole grains or starchy vegetables like brown rice, quinoa, or sweet potatoes. With this method, you can have a dinner that is well-balanced and better control how many calories you eat.

One further important piece of advice is to eat in a calm and attentive manner, taking the time to enjoy each meal and paying attention to the cues your body gives you about when it is hungry and when it is satisfied. Eating more slowly may help avoid overeating since it takes the brain around 20 minutes to notice that the stomach is full.

Keep in mind that just because you are trying to manage your portion sizes, this does not imply that you have to deprive yourself or give up all of your favorite meals. You can still eat your favorite sweets in moderation, but you should be aware of the size of the portions you eat and how they affect your daily calorie count.

Mindful eating

The practice of paying attention to both your body and the food that you are consuming while you are eating, which is referred to as "mindful eating," may be done during meals or snacks. You can better recognize the signals that tell you when you are hungry and when you have had enough to eat if you practice mindfulness and bring your attention to the food that you are currently eating. This will allow you to make more nutritious decisions regarding the food that you consume and the amount that you consume.

The following is a list of some suggestions for developing a mindful eating practice:

- *Slow down:* Eating slowly and thoughtfully may help you taste the flavor of your meal and become aware of when you have reached your maximum capacity for eating.

- *Eliminate distractions:* When you're eating, make sure you get rid of any potential distractions by turning off the television and putting away your phone. This will help you pay attention to the taste of the food and the feelings that come from eating.

- *Pay attention to your senses:* Really taste and appreciate the food that you are eating by taking your time with it. Take note of the many aromas, flavors, and textures that come with each mouthful.

- *Listen to your body:* Pay attention to the cues that your body sends you about hunger and fullness. Eat only when you are hungry and stop when you are content with the amount you have consumed.

- *Be mindful of portion sizes:* Pay attention to the serving sizes that are advised, and utilize measurement equipment like a food scale to help you remain on track with your eating plan.

- *Practice gratitude:* Try pausing for a minute to acknowledge and appreciate the sustenance that comes from the food that you eat.

If you practice mindful eating, you might change the way you feel about food and learn more about what your body needs. This might help you control how much you eat so you don't overeat and choose foods that are healthier and better for your body's health.

Hydration

Maintaining a healthy level of hydration is important for losing weight and staying healthy in general. If you want to keep hydrated, flush out toxins, and support the metabolic processes in your body, drinking a lot of water and other liquids that are low in calories is a great way to do all of those things. In addition to being a natural appetite suppressant, drinking water may also make you feel fuller. As a result, you may be able to cut down on the number of calories you consume each day, which can be beneficial to your attempts to lose weight.

In addition to water, herbal tea, green tea, and sparkling water are also examples of drinks that don't have any calories and may help you stay well-hydrated. It is important to steer clear of sugary beverages like soda and fruit juices since they contain a lot of calories and may make it difficult to lose weight.

It is essential to keep in mind that the amount of water that a person requires may change significantly based on a variety of circumstances, including the size of their body, the intensity of their activities, and the weather. A good rule of thumb is to strive to consume at least 8 cups (64 ounces) of water each day, and you should aim to consume even more water if you are physically active or live in a warm region. Keeping a water bottle with you at all times could be a good way to make sure you stay hydrated and stay on track with your goals.

Consistency

One of the most important things you can do to lose weight for good is to stick to the same diet and exercise plan. Even though it's tempting to try crash diets or intense workout programs, research shows that making small, consistent changes to your lifestyle is better in the long run.

Create a healthy eating plan that you can follow with some regularity; that will be one method to create consistency. This diet has to include a wide range of wholesome meals that are high in nutrients, and the portion sizes need to be just right. It's important to find meals that you really like and to make sure your diet can be maintained for a long time.

Setting goals that you can reach and keeping track of how you're doing are two more important parts of staying consistent. Keeping this in mind might make it easier for you to maintain your motivation and make appropriate changes. Celebrating your accomplishments along the way, no matter how small they may seem, will help you generate momentum and ensure that you stay on course.

It's important to remember that being consistent doesn't mean you've reached perfection. As long as they are part of an otherwise healthy and well-balanced life, the occasional slip-up or treat can be tolerated without fear of bad things happening. The most important thing is to get back on track and ensure that you are still making steady headway toward your desired level of weight reduction.

It is important to keep in mind that the nutritional requirements of a person might vary greatly depending on variables such as their age, gender, level of activity, and the health issues they are dealing with. If you talk to a registered dietitian or other health care professional, they can help you make a nutrition plan that is right for you.

Chapter 4

Exercise for Weight Loss: The Best Types of Exercises for Fast Results

Exercise is a key part of any plan to lose body fat because it helps burn calories, build muscle, and speed up the metabolism. On the other hand, not every kind of physical activity has the same impact on one's ability to shed pounds. There are some forms of exercise that are superior to others when it comes to the number of calories they burn and the amount of fat they help one lose. Here are some of the best ways to exercise to lose a lot of weight quickly:

High-intensity interval training (HIIT): HIIT is a popular way to work out. It involves going back and forth between short bursts of intense exercise and rest or less intense activity. The high-intensity intervals usually last anywhere from 20 to 60 seconds, and they are followed by a rest or recovery period that lasts anywhere from 10 to 60 seconds. This range depends on how fit the person is and how hard they are working out.

One of the best things about high-intensity interval training is that it may help you burn more calories in less time than steady-state cardio workouts. High-intensity interval training (HIIT) might be a good way to get a calorie deficit, which is necessary for losing weight. This form of exercise not only gets your heart rate up but also revs up your metabolism, both of which may help you burn more calories when your session is complete.

HIIT workouts can also be done with a wide range of activities, such as jogging, cycling, or even body-weight exercises like burpees or jump squats. Because of this, High-Intensity Interval Training (HIIT) is a flexible and changing type of exercise that can be changed to fit your preferences and level of fitness.

Studies have shown that high intensity interval training (HIIT) may be an effective method for reducing body fat, particularly when accompanied with a balanced diet. A study that was presented at the International Congress on Obesity and published in the International Journal of Obesity found that women who did high-intensity interval training (HIIT) three times a week for 15 weeks lost a lot more body fat than women who did steady-state cardio exercise for 15 weeks.

It is essential to keep in mind that high-intensity interval training (HIIT) is a kind of intense exercise, and thus, it may not be appropriate for everyone. Before beginning a high-intensity interval training (HIIT) program, people who are just starting out or who have health issues should check in with their primary care provider. To reduce the risk of injury, it is essential to begin your exercises at a modest level and gradually build up both the length and the intensity of your routine as time goes on.

In general, high-intensity interval training (HIIT) is an effective way to burn calories and lose weight that doesn't take up too much time. Adding high-intensity interval training (HIIT) to your exercise routine is a great way to reach your weight loss goals more quickly and improve your overall fitness and health.

Resistance Training: Resistance training, which is sometimes just called "resistance training," is an exercise that involves putting force against your own body. Its goal is to make you stronger and more durable. It is possible to do this task with the use of free weights, resistance bands, equipment, or even simply one's own body weight.

Resistance training has many benefits, such as improving overall physical performance, increasing bone density, making muscles stronger and more durable, and making it easier to gain strength. In addition to this, it may be an important factor in the process of reducing and managing one's weight.

One of the key advantages of resistance training is that it helps to grow muscle mass, which is one of the many benefits of this kind of exercise. Since muscle tissue is metabolically active, it lets you keep burning calories even when you're not actively moving around. Because you have more muscle, your resting metabolic rate may be higher. In fact, studies have shown that weight training may give your metabolism a boost that lasts for up to three days after you've finished your exercise.

In addition to helping you lose weight and keep it off, resistance training may also increase your insulin sensitivity, which is essential for effective weight reduction and maintenance. If you have more insulin sensitivity, your body will be able to use insulin more effectively. This will make it easier for glucose to get into your cells and be used as a source of energy. Insulin resistance is a disease that, if left untreated, may lead to weight gain as well as type 2 diabetes. This can be helpful in preventing insulin resistance.

You may do resistance training in a number of different ways, and the method you choose should depend on both your objectives and your personal preferences. If you are new to resistance training, it is recommended that you begin with bodyweight exercises such as push-ups, squats, and lunges. These exercises are a fantastic way to get your muscles warmed up and ready to work.

These workouts are excellent for putting on muscle, and the best part is that you don't need any special equipment to accomplish them. As you get stronger, you can make your exercises more difficult by adding weights or resistance bands. This is something you can do as you go through your strength training.

To get the most out of resistance training, you must use the right form and technique. This will help keep you from getting hurt and make sure you're working the right muscles during your workout. Think about working with a personal trainer or enrolling in a group fitness class if you are unsure of how to get started with your fitness routine. They can assist, direct you through correct form and technique, and give you a range of exercises to keep your workouts interesting and successful.

In a nutshell, resistance training is a good way to burn calories, build muscle, and improve one's physical performance overall. You will be able to reach your weight loss and fitness objectives, as well as enhance your metabolism, improve your insulin sensitivity, and become more fit if you include resistance training in your exercise program.

Cardiovascular   Exercise:

Cardiovascular exercises include jogging, cycling, and swimming. Most people just call all of these activities "cardio." This is an excellent way to improve your cardiovascular health and burn off some calories at the same time. Having said that, it is necessary to emphasize the fact that cardiovascular exercise

should not be depended on as the only type of exercise for weight reduction since it mostly burns calories during the activity itself and does not have as substantial an effect on growing muscle mass or the metabolic rate as resistance training does. Instead, resistance training should be focused on.

Having said that, including cardiovascular activity in a weight-loss regimen might still prove to be a very beneficial addition. In addition to providing a mental pick-me-up and causing the release of endorphins, exercise may help increase one's endurance and general level of physical fitness. Adults should get at least 150 minutes of cardiovascular activity per week at a moderate level or at least 75 minutes of cardiovascular exercise per week at a vigorous intensity, according to the guidelines provided by the American Heart Association.

It is essential to locate a cardiovascular workout activity that you can include in your lifestyle while also finding something that you love doing. Increasing your adherence to your workout regimen and making it more likely that you will continue to do so are two of the benefits that can be gained from doing so. Including interval training or high intensity intervals into your workout routine will help you burn more calories and improve your cardiovascular fitness in an even more significant way.

Compound Exercises: Compound exercises are a sort of strength training exercise that involves exercising many muscle groups and joints simultaneously. This type of exercise is also known as a multi-joint exercise. Unlike isolation exercises, which only work one muscle group at a time, compound exercises work many muscle groups at once. Isolation exercises concentrate on developing only one particular muscle group. Because of this, they are more effective than other methods for gaining general strength and muscular mass, and as a result, they are often used in exercise routines designed to help people shed excess pounds.

One of the most common and effective compound exercises is the squat, which entails bending at the hips and knees to lower the body until it is in the same position as when sitting in a chair, and then returning to the starting position. Squats work a lot of different muscle groups at the same time, including the quadriceps, glutes, hamstrings, and calves. The deadlift is another common kind of compound exercise. In this exercise, the legs, hips, and back all work together to raise a weight off the ground. The glutes, hamstrings, lower back, and core muscles are all worked by exercises that focus on the deadlift.

Compound exercises are not only good for growing strength and muscular mass, but they also aid in burning more calories and improving overall fitness. Compound exercises may be broken down into three categories: Since they demand more energy to do, they have the potential to improve one's heart rate and burn more calories than solitary exercises do. Also, because they work more muscle groups at once, they are good for improving both functional movement patterns and athleticism as a whole.

It is vital to pick compound exercises that target the precise muscle groups and movement patterns that you want to concentrate on when introducing compound exercises into a training program. This is because compound exercises target more than one muscle group at a time. For instance, squats and lunges are fantastic for growing leg strength as well as improving general lower body function. On the other hand, push-ups and pull-ups are wonderful for building upper body strength as well as improving core stability. To avoid injury and get the most out of the exercise, it is important to do the move correctly and with the right technique.

Circuit Training: Circuit training is a common kind of physical activity that involves completing a number of exercises in a sequence, with a minimal amount of rest in between each set of exercises. Before moving on to the next exercise, you have to do the last one for a set amount of time or a set number of times. This kind of exercise may help improve your cardiovascular endurance, help you burn calories, and help you build muscle.

A circuit training routine can include exercises that use only the person's own bodyweight or weights like dumbbells or resistance bands. A circuit's exercises might be designed to target certain muscle groups, or they can be full-body workouts that target many muscle groups all at once.

Circuit training has several advantages, one of which is that it may make effective use of one's time. You may work out a number of different muscle groups in a very short period of time if you complete a series of exercises in a sequence. Those who have hectic lives and don't have a lot of spare time to spend working out at the gym may find this to be a particularly helpful option.

Circuit training has a lot of other benefits, and it may also help you build up your cardiovascular endurance. Your heart rate remains raised for the whole workout since there is very little to no respite in between the different exercises. Your endurance and cardiovascular health may both benefit from this, as well as your cardiovascular health.

Circuit training is another good way to burn calories and lose weight. You are able to burn more calories than you would be able to with standalone workouts due to the fact that you are training many muscle groups at the same time. Also, keeping your heart rate up while you exercise will help to rev up your metabolism and keep you losing weight even after the session is over.

In general, circuit training is a sort of exercise that is not only practical but also efficient, and it may be useful for individuals of varying levels of fitness. Circuit training is a type of exercise that doesn't take a lot of time but can help you reach a number of fitness goals, such as improving your heart health, getting stronger, and lowering your body fat percentage.

It is essential to keep in mind that the sort of physical activity that will be most effective for weight reduction will be determined by factors such as the individual's preferences, current fitness level, and general health. In order to avoid being bored with your exercises and to ensure that you are pushing your body in a variety of different ways, it is essential to switch things up often. If you talk to a trained fitness expert or doctor, they may also be able to help you make an exercise plan that fits your needs and is safe and effective.

Chapter 5

Sleep and Stress Management: The Importance of Rest and Recovery for Weight Loss

A lot of individuals put all of their attention on their food and their workout routine when it comes to getting rid of excess weight. On the other hand, it's just as important to get enough sleep and rest after hard exercise if you want to reach and keep a healthy weight. The following is a list of the most significant reasons why getting enough sleep and managing stress are both essential for weight loss:

Sleep and Metabolism: Because there is a strong link between sleep and metabolism, the amount and quality of sleep we get each night may have a lot to do with whether or not we are successful at losing body fat. While we sleep, our bodies repair damaged tissues and grow new ones. They also control hormone production and the rate at which they work. This is just one of the many important things that happen to our bodies when we sleep.

One of the most significant ways in which sleep may influence one's metabolism is via the effects that it has on the hormones that regulate one's hunger. Both leptin and ghrelin are hormones that play significant roles in the regulation of appetite and fullness. The hormone ghrelin, which comes from the stomach, makes you feel hungry, while the hormone leptin, which comes from fat cells, makes you feel less hungry. The levels of the hormone leptin fall, while the levels of the hormone ghrelin rise when we don't get enough sleep. This can make you feel more hungry and less full, which can make it harder to stick to a balanced eating plan and can lead to weight gain in the long run.

It has also been shown that not getting enough sleep can change how our bodies break down carbs. This can lead to insulin resistance and a higher chance of getting type 2 diabetes. If we don't get enough sleep, our systems make less insulin and are less able to handle glucose properly, both of which may result in higher levels of blood sugar. If we don't get enough sleep, we should try to obtain at least seven hours every night.

Getting enough sleep each night is critical for the proper regulation of the stress hormone cortisol. When we don't get enough sleep, our bodies create more cortisol, which may cause inflammation and lead to a variety of health concerns, including weight gain.

To use sleep to lose weight, it's important to try to get between 7 and 9 hours of sleep every night and to stick to a regular sleep schedule. In addition, it is crucial to sleep on a bed that is comfortable for you. This could improve the quality of sleep and help the body's natural circadian rhythms work better. You might also get a better night's sleep if you don't drink coffee or alcohol in the evening, spend less time in front of screens in the hours before nightfall, and get into a routine that helps you wind down before bed.

Stress and Overeating: Since stress can make you stop eating well and make you eat too much, it can be a big reason why you gain weight or find it hard to lose it. Also, stress might make it more difficult to make progress toward your weight loss goals. Cortisol is a hormone that is secreted by our bodies in reaction to psychological or physiological stress. This response, often known as the "fight or flight" response, gets us ready to deal with the perceived danger. Cortisol may be helpful in the short term because it helps us deal with stressful situations more quickly and effectively. The problem comes up, though, when stress lasts for a long time and cortisol levels stay high for a long time. This may contribute to weight gain in addition to other health issues.

One of the ways in which stress may contribute to overeating is by causing an increase in appetite as well as a yearning for meals that are rich in calories and fat. Cortisol has been shown to cause the production of neuropeptide Y, which is a neurotransmitter that makes people hungry and makes them store fat. Also, stress can mess up the normal chemicals in our bodies that control our hunger. This can make it harder to tell when we are full or hungry, which can lead to overeating.

One further way that stress may contribute to overeating is by causing people to eat out of emotion, which can then lead to overeating. It is common for individuals to seek solace or escape from stress via the medium of food, which may result in excessive eating and weight gain for those who do so. When people eat for emotional reasons, they often choose meals that are rich in calories and fat, which may contribute to weight gain as well as other health issues.

It is very important to learn how to deal with stress well if you want to avoid these negative effects on your ability to lose weight and your health in general. Exercising, meditating, doing exercises that include deep breathing, and even talking to a counselor are all potential stress management strategies. Developing good ways to deal with stress, like being mindful, keeping a journal, or spending time in nature, may also help stop emotional eating and overeating. Spending time in nature, writing in a journal, or practicing mindfulness are all ways to do this. Since a lack of sleep may add to stress and make it more difficult to handle successfully, making obtaining enough sleep a priority is another thing that really has to be done.

Sleep and Physical Activity: Getting enough sleep is very important if you want to be physically active and lose weight. When we get enough rest, we are able to participate in more physically demanding activities because we have the energy and drive to do so. This, in turn, might help us cut back on the calories we eat and our overall body mass. On the other hand, when we're tired, we may be more likely to skip our workouts or do things that require us to sit still, both of which can cause us to gain weight.

Several studies show that people who don't get enough sleep are more likely to lead a sedentary lifestyle than those who get the recommended amount of sleep each night. For instance, a study that was published in the Journal of Sleep Research discovered that people who slept for less than six hours per night were less active during the day than those who slept for seven to eight hours per night.

This was compared to people who slept for seven to eight hours per night. According to the findings of the research, those with lower levels of physical activity had higher body mass index (BMI) scores and a greater likelihood of being overweight or obese.

Not getting enough sleep could also hurt our athletic performance. When we are tired, our reaction times, coordination, and endurance may all slow down. This makes it harder to be active and burn calories. Also, because of this, you are more likely to get hurt when you work out.

In general, getting enough sleep is very important for both losing weight and becoming more physically active. If you want to support your weight reduction objectives and increase your athletic performance, you should aim for seven to nine hours of sleep per night. If you have trouble falling or staying asleep, try to stick to a regular sleep schedule, avoid drinking coffee or alcohol in the hours before bedtime, and make your bedroom a relaxing place to sleep.

So, what can you do to prioritize rest and recovery for weight loss?

Aim for 7-9 hours of sleep per night: It is essential to one's general health and well-being, as well as weight reduction, to get an adequate amount of sleep. The National Sleep Foundation says that people need between seven and nine hours of sleep each night to function at their best during the day.

When we don't get enough sleep, our bodies may create more of the hormone cortisol, which is linked to both increased stress and increased body fat. Not getting enough sleep can also throw off the balance of hormones that control hunger. This results in an increase in the hormone that causes hunger (ghrelin), and a reduction in the hormone that causes fullness (leptin). This may lead to excessive eating, which in turn may play a role in the development of weight gain.

In addition, not getting enough sleep may result in lower levels of energy, which makes it more difficult to participate in activities that require physical movement. Exercise is a key part of losing weight because it helps you burn calories and build muscle. Being well rested makes it more likely that we will have the energy and motivation to exercise, which in turn makes it easier to lose weight.

To make sleep a top priority, you need to get into good sleeping habits, which are often called "sleep hygiene." Setting a regular sleep schedule, staying away from stimulating activities like electronics and exercise before bed, sleeping in a calm place, and not drinking coffee or alcohol in the hours before bedtime are all possible parts of this strategy.

Getting enough sleep is an important part of both losing weight and maintaining your health in general. In order to assist your efforts to lose weight, you should aim to get between 7 and 9 hours of sleep each night and develop appropriate sleeping habits.

Practice stress management techniques: Managing stress well is an important part of getting and staying healthy and happy, and it can also help a lot with weight loss. Cortisol is a hormone that is produced by our bodies in response to stress. This hormone is associated with an increased appetite as well as a desire for meals that are rich in calories and fat. This may, over time, lead to an increase in weight as well as difficulties in maintaining a healthy weight loss. Because of this, it is important to do some kind of stress management practice to help keep cortisol levels in check and lessen the negative effects of stress on the body.

Meditation is a way to deal with stress that involves focusing on your breathing or something else in your environment, like a candle or a mantra. Recent research suggests that regular meditation may lower cortisol levels, improve mood, and make people healthier overall. Choose a place that is free from distractions and silent, where you won't be disturbed, then sit in a comfortable position with your eyes closed and practice meditation there.

Maintain your concentration on your breathing while letting your ideas come and go without evaluating them or attaching yourself to them in any way. It is possible to begin your practice with as little as a few minutes each day and then progressively expand the amount of time you spend doing it over time.

Yoga, which involves a combination of different physical postures, different breathing exercises, and meditation, is an additional method that is useful in managing stress. Yoga, like meditation, has been shown to lower levels of the stress hormone cortisol and improve mood. Yoga may also help you get stronger and more flexible, which can make you more active and help you lose weight.

Breathing exercises that focus on a slow and steady inhale and exhale are another method that is both straightforward and efficient for managing stress. When we are under a lot of pressure, our breathing has a tendency to become shallow and fast, which may make our emotions of worry and tension much worse. Deep breathing exercises may help regulate breathing and calm the nervous system, which can lead to a feeling of calmness and relaxation. In order to perfect the art of deep breathing, you should choose a comfortable position, shut your eyes, and then take long, slow breaths in via your nose. After holding your breath for a few seconds, exhale softly through your lips. Continue to suppress your breathing for a few more seconds. Continue this cycle a few times while bringing your attention to the feeling of your breath traveling in and out of your body.

Other methods of relieving stress include spending time in natural settings, participating in creative pursuits such as making music or art, and cultivating meaningful relationships with those who are important to you. Finding ways to deal with your stress that work for you and using them every day will help you lose weight and manage your stress. It is crucial to discover strategies that work for you and integrate them.

Take rest days: You need rest days in your exercise schedule so that your body can recover from the physical stress that exercise puts on it and heal itself. Taking a day or two off between workouts can help you feel less tired, prevent injuries, and help you do better in your next workout overall.

As you exercise, microscopic rips occur in your muscles, and these tears need time to mend and repair before they can be used again. This process, called "muscle recovery," is important for getting stronger and more durable because it helps the muscles rebuild and repair themselves after being used. Your muscles may not have enough time to heal if you don't get enough rest, which can result in muscular fatigue, discomfort, and a drop in performance if you don't get enough rest.

Your body needs a break from the mental and physical strains of exercise just as much as it needs a break from the exercises themselves. This could help reduce stress, improve your mood, and give you more energy and motivation for future workouts.

It is essential to keep in mind that a day of rest does not always imply that the individual will accomplish nothing at all. On the days when you are supposed to be resting, you are still able to take part in some mild forms of physical exercise. For example, you may go for a stroll, do yoga, or stretch. This may improve blood flow and make it easier for your muscles to heal without putting too much strain on your body.

If you want to get the most out of your workout regimen, you should give yourself at least one or two days off per week to relax. This could change, though, depending on your fitness goals, your current level of fitness, and the activity you are doing. It is essential to pay attention to your body and make necessary adjustments to your routine in accordance with what it tells you to do in order to get the proper amount of rest and recuperation.

You can help support your attempts to lose weight and develop a healthy lifestyle that is sustainable if you make rest and recovery a priority in your life.

Chapter 6

Hydration: Why Water Is Key to Losing Weight and Maintaining Good Health

The ability to stay hydrated is essential to one's general health and well-being, and it also plays an important part in the process of shedding unwanted pounds. Water is needed for digestion, absorption, and transport of nutrients, as well as for controlling body temperature and getting rid of waste. Water is also needed to keep waste products from building up in the body. These processes may be thrown off kilter when we are dehydrated, which can result in a variety of unpleasant health issues like constipation, kidney stones, and even kidney failure.

Not only is staying hydrated important for keeping your body running normally, but it also helps a lot when you're trying to lose weight. It's been shown that drinking water before and during meals might help you feel fuller on less food, which ultimately results in fewer calories ingested overall. This is because drinking water makes the stomach grow, which gives you a feeling of being full and makes you feel less hungry. In fact, research has shown that those who drink water before a meal end up consuming fewer calories overall than those who don't drink water before meals.

Consuming water on a regular basis might also assist in speeding up the metabolism. According to the findings of a research article that was published in the Journal of Clinical Endocrinology and Metabolism, healthy people who drank 500 milliliters (about 17 ounces) of water saw a 30% boost in their metabolic rate. Ten minutes after drinking the water, this effect started to show up, and it lasted for more than an hour. When the body is well hydrated, it is better able to do things like break down fat into energy.

Another advantage of drinking enough water is that it may help minimize the amount of water that is retained in the body. This problem, called "water retention," can cause swelling and a temporary weight gain. When the body is already dehydrated, it may hold on to water to keep from getting even more dehydrated. This can lead to bloating and puffiness. On the other hand, when the body is well hydrated, it has a lower propensity to retain more water than it needs to.

Even though water is the best choice for hydration, it is crucial to know that other drinks and meals may also contribute to overall hydration levels. This is something to keep in mind. On the other hand, it is essential to choose drinks that have a small amount of added sugar and calories, such as black tea or coffee that has not been sweetened or flavored water that does not contain added sugar. Fruits and vegetables, which contain a lot of water, may also help keep the body at the right level of hydration.

Getting enough water every day might also help you lose weight. Our bodies have the ability to confuse thirst with hunger when we are dehydrated, which may cause us to consume more food than we truly need. By maintaining a healthy level of hydration, we can avoid getting too thirsty and eating too much. Drinking water before meals may also help us feel satisfied more quickly, which can result in a reduction in the total quantity of food that we take in.

Keeping ourselves well-hydrated not only helps us get rid of extra body fat, but it also helps us stay healthy in general. Getting enough water helps our bodies get rid of toxins, which may make it less likely that we will get long-term illnesses like cancer and heart disease. In addition to these benefits, it helps to maintain the healthy appearance of our skin, and it may even boost our mood and cognitive performance.

When it comes to hydration, it is essential to keep in mind that not all liquids are created equal in terms of their hydrating potential. Since caffeine and alcohol can make us lose water, it's important to drink enough water to stay hydrated. Also, sugary beverages like soda and juice may add extra calories to our meals, which is another reason why it is ideal to choose water as our beverage whenever possible.

Aim to drink at least eight glasses of water every day to make sure you're getting enough water. However, you may need to drink even more water if you're doing hard physical work or traveling to a hotter place. If you want to avoid being dehydrated, it is important that you pay attention to the signs that your body sends you when it is thirsty and that you drink water regularly throughout the day. Getting enough water can help you lose weight and keep your health in good shape.

It goes without saying that being hydrated is critical for one's general health and well-being, as well as for successful weight reduction. If you drink water before meals, it can help you consume fewer calories overall, and maintaining a healthy level of hydration may help speed up your metabolism and cut down on the amount of fluid you retain. Try to drink at least 8 glasses (64 ounces) of water every day, as well as other low-calorie drinks and meals that are high in water. This will help you stay hydrated overall.

Chapter 7

Superfoods: Natural Ways to Boost Your Metabolism and Promote Weight Loss

Foods that are high in nutrients and are considered to have a variety of positive effects on one's health are referred to as "superfoods." These meals are full of vitamins, minerals, antioxidants, and other healthy foods that may help you lose weight and speed up your metabolism.

Here is a list of well-known superfoods that can help you lose weight:

Berries: Berries have a low calorie count and a high fiber content, both of which may help you feel full for extended periods of time. Berries can be found in almost any grocery store. They also include a high concentration of antioxidants, which have been shown to lessen the effects of inflammation and improve health in general. There are many delicious berry selections available, but some of the best ones include blueberries, raspberries, strawberries, and blackberries.

- *Greens*: Greens with Leaves Spinach, kale, and collard greens are examples of leafy greens that are rich in fiber, have a relatively low number of calories, and are excellent sources of vitamin and mineral content. These greens have chemicals that may help manage blood sugar levels, decrease inflammation, and improve digestion, all of which are benefits of eating them.

- *Avocado:* Since avocados are so rich in potassium, fiber, and heart-healthy fats, they are an excellent addition to any diet that focuses on reducing body fat. Avocado has both healthy fats and fiber, both of which may help manage digestion and blood sugar levels. The good fats in avocado can help you feel full longer, while the fiber can help regulate blood sugar levels.

- *Chia Seeds:* Chia seeds are a great source of fiber and omega-3 fatty acids, two things that may help reduce inflammation and improve heart health. Chia Seeds These little seeds have the ability to reabsorb water, which helps them maintain their ability to keep you feeling full for extended lengths of time.

- *Quinoa:* Quinoa is a grain that is high in protein and is also strong in fiber and other minerals. Quinoa is known as a superfood. Because it can help control blood sugar levels, reduce inflammation, and make you feel fuller, it is a great addition to any diet that focuses on losing weight.

- *Green Tea:* Green tea is a natural source of caffeine and antioxidants, all of which may aid in stimulating metabolism and supporting weight reduction when consumed regularly. It also has parts that help reduce inflammation and improve brain function, so it can be used for more than one thing.

- *Greek Yogurt:* Since it is both rich in protein and low in calories, Greek yogurt is an excellent supplement to a diet that focuses on weight reduction and should be consumed regularly. It may help you feel full, keep your blood sugar levels in check, and help your digestive system work better.

It is essential to emphasize that despite the fact that the items on this list may be advantageous for weight reduction, they should only be consumed as part of a healthy, well-balanced diet and should not be relied on as the only method for shedding excess pounds. When adding new items to your diet, it is essential to take into account any unique dietary limitations or allergies you may have.

Chapter 8

Intermittent Fasting: The Benefits of Fasting and How to Incorporate It into Your Life

"Intermittent fasting" is a common way to lose weight that involves alternating times when you eat with times when you don't eat or drink anything. It is not a diet in the traditional sense; rather, it is a method of eating that entails reducing the number of calories you consume at specified times of the day. There are several techniques to intermittent fasting, the most prominent of which are the 16/8 method, the 5:2 method, and alternate-day fasting. Nevertheless, intermittent fasting may be done in a variety of other ways as well.

One of the most well-known and often used approaches to fasting is called the 16:8 technique, which involves alternating periods of eating and not eating for 16 hours. The day is broken up into two parts: an eating window and a fasting window. This is done so that you may lose weight. During the eating window, you eat all of your daily calories. During the fasting window, you don't drink anything but water, black coffee, or other non-caloric liquids.

By reducing the total number of calories you eat each day, the 16/8 approach may help you lose weight. This is done by giving yourself less time each day to eat. This is due to the fact that it might be difficult to consume the same amount of calories in a shorter period of time, particularly if you generally consume a lot of meals that are rich in calories or processed.

The 16:8 strategy of intermittent fasting is associated with a variety of possible health advantages, in addition to its effectiveness in fostering weight reduction. For instance, studies show that it may help increase insulin sensitivity, which may lead to a reduced chance of developing type 2 diabetes. Also, it might be able to help lower blood pressure, reduce inflammation, and improve brain function.

Establishing a regular pattern of eating and fasting is essential if you want to successfully implement the 16/8 approach into your lifestyle. This entails giving yourself a predetermined window of time each day—eight hours—during which you will eat all of your daily calories, and then going without food for the other sixteen hours of the day. Picking an eating window that is conducive to one's daily routine and overall way of life is something that a lot of individuals find to be of great assistance. If you have a job that requires you to be there from 9 to 5, for instance, you may decide to eat anytime between noon and eight o'clock at night.

It is essential to keep in mind that the 16/8 approach may not be appropriate for everyone. Before trying intermittent fasting, people with certain health problems, like diabetes, should talk to a qualified medical professional about their plans. Also, it's important to pay attention to the signs your body gives you and change your fasting schedule accordingly. During your fast, if you feel symptoms like lightheadedness, dizziness, or extreme hunger, you may need to change the length of your fasting window or the time you eat.

The 5:2 method, also known as the Fast Diet, is a form of intermittent fasting that entails eating normally for five days out of the week and then restricting calorie intake to between 500 and 600 calories on two days that are not consecutive. This type of fasting can help individuals lose weight by reducing their overall calorie intake. This method has become well-known as a way to lose weight and improve health. Dr. Michael Mosley is credited with making the method well-known and bringing it to the forefront.

During the two days when participants aren't allowed to eat, they usually eat just two small meals with a total of 500 to 600 calories. Most of the time, these meals have a low amount of carbs and a high amount of protein and fiber to help you feel full and stop you from getting hungry. Individuals are free to consume as many calories as they like for the remaining five days of the diet, however, it is strongly advised that they stick to a nutritious and well-balanced eating plan during the whole diet.

The fact that the 5:2 approach provides for some leeway in terms of eating habits while still providing the benefits of intermittent fasting is among the most significant advantages offered by this strategy. People might find it easier to stick to the diet if they only cut back on calories two days a week instead of using stricter methods that require them to fast every day or keep track of their calories.

Several pieces of research have shown that the 5:2 approach is an effective way to lose weight. In a pilot study that was later published in the International Journal of Obesity, researchers found that obese participants who followed the 5:2 diet lost more weight and body fat than those who followed a daily calorie restriction diet. This was the case despite the fact that both groups consumed the same total number of calories. Several studies have also shown that fasting for shorter periods of time at regular intervals may help increase insulin sensitivity, reduce inflammation, and improve overall health indices.

It is essential to keep in mind, however, that the 5:2 technique may not be appropriate for every person. Before making big changes to your diet, you should always talk to a doctor or other health professional. It is possible that it is not ideal for persons who have a history of disordered eating, and it is also highly recommended that one do so.

In a nutshell, the 5:2 technique is an intermittent fasting plan that involves eating normally for five days and then cutting calories to between 500 and 600 per day for two days that are not consecutive. This strategy might help you reach your weight loss goals, and it might also help you maintain the benefits of intermittent fasting while giving you more freedom with your food choices.

Alternate-day fasting is a type of intermittent fasting in which you eat normally one day and then fast the next. As a method for shedding extra pounds, it is also known as the "ADF" diet and has recently seen a rise in its level of acceptance. Alternate-day fasting is a method of weight loss in which one day of the week is spent consuming fewer calories than usual (hence the name), while the other five days of the week are spent eating normally. The goal of this method is to create a caloric deficit, which can then be made up for by eating more than usual on the non-

People who do alternate-day fasting usually eat between 500 and 600 calories or less on the days they have to fast. One way to meet your daily calorie limit is to eat a light meal in the evening. Another way is to eat your daily calorie limit in several smaller meals spread out throughout the day. The specific order in which meals are consumed on fasting days might vary from person to person based on their tastes and the way they live their lives.

People can eat as usual on days when they don't have to fast, but it's important to remember that eating too much can still make a person gain weight. In order to promote one's general health and sense of well-being, it is important to concentrate on eating meals that are complete and include nutrients. Some people may find that, because of the habits they've formed while fasting, even when they're not restricting their food intake, they still eat less than usual on days when they're not fasting.

The practice of fasting every other day may have health advantages in a number of different areas. Because this strategy may help create a calorie deficit over time, one of the most important benefits is weight loss. Also, it might make the body more sensitive to insulin, which could help control blood sugar levels and lower the risk of getting type 2 diabetes. Alternate day fasting has also been proposed, based on the findings of a few studies, to be able to enhance indicators of cardiovascular health, such as blood pressure and cholesterol levels.

On the other hand, the practice of fasting every other day may not be appropriate for all individuals. It is possible that those who have specific medical issues, like diabetes, should not do it, and individuals who have a history of eating disorders may find it tough. Before starting a new way of eating or fasting, it is important to talk to a health professional.

In general, fasting every other day may be a good way to reach your weight loss goals and improve your health as a whole. It needs a certain amount of dedication and discipline, but it may allow flexibility in eating patterns and may lead to improvements in eating habits that are sustainable.

Alternating periods of abstinence from food consumption with periods of consumption is the fundamental tenet of the diet strategy known as intermittent fasting. Intermittent fasting can be done in different ways, and each way has its own strategy and possible health benefits. Overall, intermittent fasting has been linked to a number of possible benefits, such as weight loss and better health in general.

The most well-known benefit of intermittent fasting is probably that it helps people lose weight. Intermittent fasting may help you lose weight by creating a calorie deficit, which is needed for weight loss, and by limiting your calorie intake during fasting periods. Several studies have also shown that intermittent fasting may be more effective than standard calorie-restricted diets for both short-term and long-term weight loss and maintenance.

It has also been shown that intermittent fasting may make the body more sensitive to insulin, which is important for controlling blood sugar and lowering the risk of getting type 2 diabetes. Periods of fasting have been shown to help lower insulin resistance and enhance glucose absorption by the cells of the body, both of which may lead to improvements in the ability to keep blood sugar under control.

In addition to this, research has shown that those who practice intermittent fasting have lower levels of inflammation throughout their bodies. Chronic inflammation may play a role in the development of long-term illnesses like cancer, diabetes, and heart disease. Intermittent fasting may help lower the risk of some diseases by lowering inflammation, which may be a factor in how they develop.

Some research has shown that going on fasts for shorter periods of time may enhance cognitive performance and lower the chance of developing neurological disorders like Parkinson's disease and Alzheimer's disease. Brain-derived neurotrophic factor (BDNF) levels go up when you don't eat for a while. Fasting also helps the brain make new neurons. BDNF is a protein that plays an important part in learning and memory. Fasting may be beneficial for those who want to lose weight.

As you start implementing intermittent fasting into your lifestyle, it is imperative that you pay attention to how your body reacts and listen to what it has to say. During fasting, it's important to stay hydrated and not eat too much when you can. Some people may feel bad things like hunger, irritability, and tiredness when they are fasting. Because of this, it is very important to start slowly and make changes as needed.

Intermittent fasting may be a good way for people to lose weight and improve their overall health. It is important to note, however, that intermittent fasting may not be right for everyone and should be done carefully, especially by people with certain health problems. When beginning any kind of new diet or fitness routine, it is usually a good idea to talk things over with a qualified medical practitioner.

Chapter 9

Sustainable Weight Loss: How to Maintain Your Results and Live a Healthy Lifestyle

Many people who want to improve their health and well-being as a whole make reaching their ideal weight one of their main goals. Even though these goals may be possible, it may be hard to maintain the benefits of losing weight quickly and living a healthy lifestyle. Rapid weight reduction is not the same as sustainable weight loss, since sustainable weight loss involves not only maintaining a healthy weight but also living a healthy lifestyle over the long term. It means making changes to your life that are good for you and can be maintained over time. These changes should also be easy to fit into your everyday life. The following are some suggestions on how to accomplish long-term weight reduction and keep the results:

Set Realistic Goals

It is essential to understand that losing weight is a slow process that calls for patience and persistence on the part of the dieter. You'll have a better chance of reaching your ultimate weight loss goals and a clear path to get there if you set goals that are attainable and within your reach. Here are some pointers to keep in mind while attempting to develop objectives that are both realistic and sustainable for weight loss:

- *Consult a Healthcare Professional:* They can look at your health as a whole and help you set goals that are realistic, taking into account your body type, lifestyle, and any health problems you already have.

- *Set short-term and long-term goals:* Setting both short-term and long-term goals is very important if you want to lose weight successfully. Goals for the week or month are examples of short-term objectives, and objectives for the year or longer are examples of long-term objectives. This way of keeping track of your progress will help you stay motivated throughout the process.

- *Use the SMART Goal Method:* The SMART technique stands for the Specific, Measurable, Achievable, Relevant, and Time-Bound goal setting method. With the help of this plan, you can make sure that your goals are clear, measurable, and, most importantly, achievable in the time you have. A SMART goal may be phrased as follows: "I will lose one pound every week by lowering the amount of calories I consume by 500 per day for the next three months."

- *Be realistic:* When you establish a goal to lose weight, one of the most important things you can do is make sure that you are being honest with yourself about what you can really do. It is unrealistic to expect to shed 20 pounds in a single month or to go from being a couch potato to running a marathon in a single week. It is important to have a realistic outlook on the amount of weight you can reduce and the length of time it will take to accomplish your objectives.

- *Focus on Healthy Habits:* Instead of only trying to lose extra body fat, you should work on developing healthy habits like staying active, eating well, and getting enough sleep. These behaviors will help you lose weight in a healthy way that won't stop working for you, and they'll make it easier to keep the results you've achieved.

For long-term success, it's important to set goals for losing weight that are both realistic and attainable. You'll have a better chance of reaching your ultimate weight loss goals and a clear path to get there if you set goals that are attainable and within your reach. It is very important to talk to a trained doctor, come up with both short-term and long-term goals, use the SMART goal technique, keep a positive attitude, and focus on healthy behaviors.

Make Healthy Food Choices

It's not enough to just cut back on calories; you should also try to eat more foods that are high in nutrients. These foods will give your body the energy and nutrients it needs to work as well as possible. Here are some helpful hints to keep in mind when it comes to selecting nutritious foods:

- *Eat plenty of fruits and vegetables:* Fruits and vegetables are excellent sources of a variety of nutrients, including vitamins, minerals, fiber, and antioxidants. During each meal, you should make it a goal to fill up at least half of your plate with fruits and vegetables.

- *Choose whole grains:* Brown rice, quinoa, and whole-wheat bread are examples of grains that are still in their whole form. Whole grains are high in fiber, which may help you feel full and satisfied after eating them. Also, they are a great source of important minerals like iron and the B vitamins. In addition, they are an excellent source of essential minerals such as iron and the B vitamins.

- *Choose lean protein:* Select lean protein sources such as chicken, fish, beans, and tofu when looking for ways to include protein in your diet. Even though these meals don't have a lot of calories, they are high in protein, which helps you feel full and satisfied even though they aren't very big.

- *Include healthy fats:* Fats are an essential element of a healthy diet, but it is crucial to pick the proper types of fats. It is essential that you include nutritious fats in your diet. Make an effort to consume more healthy fats, such as those that may be found in nuts, seeds, avocados, and olive oil.

- *Avoid processed foods:* Steer clear of processed foods since they often include a large amount of calories, sugar, and fat that are harmful for you. Instead, commit as much of your eating as you can to foods that are whole and unadulterated.

- *Limit sugary drinks and snacks:* Sugary beverages like soda and juice may add a lot of unnecessary calories to your diet, and they don't provide any nutritional advantages. Restrict your intake of these beverages and foods. Choose a healthy beverage instead, such as water, unsweetened tea, or sparkling water. When it comes to choosing snacks, choose nutritious alternatives like fruits, vegetables, nuts, and seeds.

Keep in mind that just because you are making changes to your diet to improve your health does not mean that you have to give up eating the things you like the most. It's all about finding that happy medium between excess and deprivation. You can have a slice of pizza or a piece of cake, but you should watch how much you eat and how many times a week you do unhealthy things. While trying to lose weight in a way that won't be temporary, one of the most important things to do is to include healthy behaviors in their daily routine.

Exercise Regularly

Consistent exercise is important for getting and staying at a healthy weight, as well as for your general health. When you exercise, you can burn calories, build muscle, and speed up your metabolism. Also, it makes it less likely that you will get diseases like heart disease, diabetes, or cancer in the future.

Most days of the week, you should try to do at least half an hour of moderately intense physical activity. In the event that you find it necessary to do so, you may divide it up into many shorter periods spread out throughout the day. Take, for instance, going for a brisk walk after each meal for ten minutes or working out for a few minutes during your lunch break. All of these options are great ways to get more exercise. Make it a consistent part of your routine so that it becomes second nature to you. This is the most crucial thing.

You can choose from a wide range of physical activities that help you keep or improve your health and lose extra weight. If you've never worked out before, walking is a fantastic activity to begin with since it doesn't require any equipment. It is gentle on your joints, it does not call for any specialized equipment, and it can be done almost anywhere. As your fitness level goes up, you'll be able to gradually pick up the pace of your run and go farther.

Jogging, cycling, swimming, dancing, and participating in aerobics programs are some examples of other forms of cardiovascular exercise. These exercises can help you burn calories and improve your heart rate, so get involved! Pick something that you take pleasure in doing, and make it a part of your daily routine as much as you can. This will help you stay motivated and get into the habit of being physically active every day.

In addition to being essential for general health, strength training is a vital component in successful weight reduction. It helps you gain muscle mass, which in turn speeds up your metabolism and causes you to burn more calories even when you're not actively doing anything. Squats, lunges, push-ups, and planks are just some of the exercises that may be performed with either free weights, resistance bands, or just your own bodyweight. Make it a goal to participate in some kind of strength training at least twice a week.

Always keep in mind that any kind of physical activity is preferable to none. Try to keep moving as much as you can throughout the day, even if you can't commit to a complete 30-minute session of exercise at one time. Use the stairs instead of the elevator, park farther away from your destination, or go for a walk while you're on your break. All of these are great ways to get more exercise. Every little bit helps you get closer to your overall goal, and it might help you as you try to lose weight.

Manage Stress

Stress is an unavoidable part of life, but it can make it hard to lose body fat. In response to emotional or physical stress, your body makes the hormone cortisol. This hormone has been linked to a bigger appetite, a greater desire for meals high in sugar and fat, and the buildup of extra fat around the abdomen. Because of this, it's important to learn how to deal with stress well if you want to lose weight in a healthy way.

There are many different methods available to you that may be used to deal with the stress in your life. Regular exercise has been shown to improve mood and lower cortisol levels. As a result, it is one of the therapies that has the highest success rate. At a level that is moderately challenging, physical activity should be conducted on most days of the week for at least half an hour. You are free to choose any kind of physical exercise that appeals to your sense of fun, such as jogging, walking, dancing, or swimming.

Meditation with an awareness of the present moment is an additional stress-relieving method that works well. Paying attention in a non-judgmental way to the happenings in the here and now is an essential component in the practice of mindfulness. The practice of mindfulness meditation has been demonstrated to increase sleep quality and immunological function, in addition to lowering levels of stress, anxiety, and depression, as uncovered by several research studies. You can get help with meditation through apps like Headspace and Calm, or you can find guided meditations online.

Another helpful strategy for stress management is participating in yoga classes. It helps reduce stress and improve overall health by combining ways to relax with physical movement. The goal of the practice is to make the person more aware of their breathing. The benefits of yoga may be felt even after practicing for just a short period of time each day.

Breathing exercises that focus on increasing the depth of your breath are another helpful method for managing stress. In these, the breaths are taken slowly and deeply, and the exhalation is done in a controlled manner. This assists in lowering the heart rate and releasing stress that has built up throughout the body. You may try a simple method such as taking a breath in for the count of four, holding it for the count of seven, and then releasing it for the count of eight.

Lastly, taking part in a relaxing activity like a hobby could be another good way to deal with stress. This may be anything that you love doing and find relaxing, such as reading, crocheting, gardening, or listening to music. Consider the things that make you feel the most at ease.. Make it a point to give yourself time every day to relax and unwind by partaking in a pastime of your own.

In addition to these measures, one of the most essential things you can do to manage your stress is make sure you are getting enough sleep. Your goal should be to get between seven and nine hours of sleep each night. Cortisol levels may go up when you don't get enough sleep, which makes it harder to deal with stress and stick to healthy habits. Sleep deprivation also makes it more difficult to concentrate and remember things.

Stay Accountable

Maintaining a sense of accountability during the weight reduction process is a key component of achieving long-term success. When you have someone else with whom you can discuss your achievements, it might be easier for you to maintain your motivation and keep your attention on your objectives. Keeping one's word may be done in a few different ways, including the following:

- *Find a Friend or Family Member:* Having a friend or family member who is also working on their weight reduction goals may be an incredible assistance. You can keep each other uplifted and motivated by sharing your successes and struggles, as well as the ways in which you're working through them.

- *Join a Weight Loss Group:* There are a lot of weight loss groups available, both online and in-person, so why not join one? The people who belong to these groups make up a community in which they all try to reach similar goals. They are able to provide assistance in the form of advice, encouragement, and accountability.

- *Work with a personal trainer or nutritionist:* Working with a personal trainer or nutritionist can help you set goals that are realistic and come up with a plan to reach those goals. In addition to this, they are able to provide direction and support to you all the way through your weight reduction journey.

- *Use technology:* There are a number of applications and websites available that may assist you in tracking your progress and remaining responsible. Using these tools will assist you in keeping track of the calories you consume, the amount of activity you get, and the amount of weight you lose. In addition, they may serve as a reminder of important details and a source of inspiration to keep moving forward.

- *Keep a Food and Exercise Journal:* Documenting the foods you eat and the exercises you do in a journal might assist you in holding yourself responsible. Keep a food and exercise journal to keep track of everything you consume and how much activity you get each day. This will help you see how far you've come and figure out where you might need to make changes.

In short, if you want to lose weight and keep it off, you need to keep your sense of responsibility. Finding a friend or family member to hold you responsible, joining a weight loss group, working with a professional, making use of technology, or keeping a diary are all great methods to remain accountable, and all of these things may help you reach your weight reduction objectives.

Avoid Fad Diets

Many people are tempted to try fad diets because they promise rapid and significant weight reduction with little to no effort on their part. But they can't be kept up indefinitely, and if you do them for a long time, it could be bad for your health. Trendy diets often involve cutting out whole food groups or eating very few calories. This may result in vitamin shortages as well as other health concerns.

There are a lot of diet fads out there, and many of them are based on assertions that lack supporting data or on older research. For example, some fad diets say that certain foods or minerals are "toxic" or "bad" for your health, even though there is no scientific evidence to support these claims. Some fad diets could advertise weight reduction pills or other goods that haven't been scientifically shown to be effective or that might even be harmful.

On the other hand, a method of weight reduction that is sustainable emphasizes making adjustments to one's lifestyle that are beneficial to one's health and that one can continue to practice over time. This involves consuming a diet that is well-balanced and contains a wide range of foods that are rich in nutrients, such as fruits, vegetables, whole grains, lean proteins, and healthy fats. In addition, you need to be physically active on a regular basis, learn how to deal with stress well, and get enough sleep.

Focusing on the science behind weight loss is one way to make it less likely that you'll fall for a fad diet. A plan for long-term weight loss should be based on good ideas about how to eat and should be supported by information from reputable scientific studies. Working with a licensed dietician or another health expert can help you make a plan to lose weight that fits your needs and goals.

In summary, despite the fact that fad diets may encourage you to believe that they can help you lose weight rapidly and without much effort, these diets are not sustainable and may even be dangerous to your health. Instead, you should concentrate on making positive adjustments to your lifestyle that you will be able to keep up over the long term. This will help you lose weight in a way that is not only sustainable but will also enhance your overall health and well-being.

Making changes to your lifestyle that are healthy and can be kept up over time are important parts of a plan to lose weight that is meant to last. Managing stress, making appropriate food choices, exercising frequently, staying responsible, and avoiding fad diets are all necessary components of this process. Setting objectives that are attainable is also important. If you follow these tips, you'll be able to lose weight and keep it off so you can live a healthy life.

Chapter 10

Common Obstacles and How to Overcome Them: Tips for Sticking to Your Weight Loss Goals

Losing weight is a journey, and just like any other journey, it comes with its share of obstacles. When people want to lose weight, the following are some of the most common problems they face:

Lack of motivation

It might be challenging to overcome an insufficiency of motivation, which is a typical difficulty in the process of weight reduction. A lot of individuals begin their quest to lose weight with a lot of excitement, but after a few weeks or months, they lose steam and find it tough to continue with their good habits. This may happen for a variety of reasons, including a lack of fast results, boredom with the same exercise regimen or healthy diet plan, or a busy and demanding lifestyle.

It is essential, however, that you constantly remind yourself of the motivations that led you to begin your path toward a healthier weight in the first place. These objectives, whether they are to enhance your health, raise your confidence, or make you feel better about yourself, may offer a sense of purpose and the incentive to continue with your healthy habit routines. Put your objectives in writing and post them in a prominent location, such as on the front of your refrigerator or the mirror in your bathroom, so that you are constantly reminded of the reason you began.

Another way to stay motivated is to ask for help from people you care about, such as family and friends. Throughout your path to a healthier weight, it may be quite helpful to have people who will encourage and support you along the way. Discuss your objectives with a close friend or member of your family who can both support you and hold you accountable for achieving them. You may also get motivation by reading success stories of other individuals who have lost the desired amount of weight and maintained their achievement. Joining a community in person or online that helps people lose weight may make them feel like they belong and give them motivation to keep going.

Change things up if you feel that you are becoming uninterested in your normal workout regimen or the foods that you eat to be healthy. Experiment with a new form of physical activity or a different style of training class, such as hiking, swimming, or dancing. Make an effort to eat more healthfully by attempting new dishes or exploring a wider variety of fruits and vegetables. Keeping your journey to a healthier weight interesting and enjoyable is important for maintaining motivation.

Last but not least, if you lead a hectic and stressful lifestyle, it could be difficult for you to make your health and weight reduction objectives a priority in your life. Yet, it is necessary to schedule time in your schedule for yourself and your wellbeing. This might be as simple as going for a stroll during your lunch break or doing a little exercise in the morning before you go to work. You can stay motivated and on track with your goals by giving yourself a high priority when it comes to self-care and ways to deal with stress, like meditation or deep breathing.

Emotional Eating

Emotional eating is when people use food to deal with their feelings instead of as a source of energy for their bodies. This is a common reason why people can't lose weight. Stress, boredom, anxiety, sadness, or even happiness are just a few of the emotions and situations that can lead to emotional eating. It might be challenging to keep under control, but there are methods to get over this obstacle.

Finding the causes that lead to emotional eating is the first step in developing a solution to the problem of overeating due to negative emotions. Maintaining a food diary will assist you in keeping track of your eating patterns and recognizing tendencies that may contribute to emotional eating. You may keep a journal in which you record the foods you consume, the times at which you consume them, and how you feel before and after eating them. This will assist you in gaining an understanding of the emotional triggers that you are susceptible to, as well as in formulating ways to avoid those triggers.

Finding healthy methods to deal with one's stress and one's negative emotions is another method for overcoming the problem of eating when one is emotionally upset. This may be accomplished by activities such as exercise, meditation, yoga, or deep breathing, or through a pastime that is calming. Participating in these activities may assist you in lowering your stress levels and enhancing your mood, both of which may, in turn, lessen the emotional hunger that you feel like you need to satisfy by eating.

It is essential to establish an atmosphere that encourages healthy eating. This requires making a conscious effort to steer clear of the temptation to fill one's kitchen with junk food and instead focus on wholesome meal preparation and consumption. When you do feel the want to eat because of your emotions, make an effort to go for nutritious snacks like fruits, veggies, or nuts when you do so.

In addition, reaching out for support from other people may be another beneficial strategy for getting over emotional eating. You may conquer emotional eating and stay committed to your weight loss objectives by working with a therapist or joining a support group for people who are losing weight. These options can give you with the skills and resources you need.

In summary, overcoming emotional eating involves a mix of self-awareness, healthy coping methods, and the creation of an environment. You will be able to effectively overcome emotional eating and achieve weight loss that is sustainable if you take the time to recognize your triggers, locate healthy methods to handle stress, and seek assistance when you feel you need it.

Busy schedule

When someone is always on the go, it's easy to put their health on the back burner, particularly when it comes to making sure they eat well and get enough exercise on a regular basis. There are, however, ways to get past this obstacle and keep working towards your weight loss goals.

One of the most effective ways to deal with a busy schedule is to put your health first. This involves making time in your schedule for physical activity on a regular basis, just as you would for any other appointment. You have the option of scheduling your appointment either before you start work, during your lunch break, or after you finish for the day. It's important to find a form of exercise that you enjoy, because that will make it much easier for you to stick to the routine over time. There are several ways to include physical activity into a hectic schedule, including the following:

- Taking a vigorous stroll during your lunch break

- Watching a short home exercise video in the morning or evening before going to work.
- By enrolling in a fitness class that is convenient for you, such as an early morning yoga session or an after-work spin class, you may get in shape.

Not only is it important to make time for physical activity, but it is also important to plan meals ahead of time. When you're pressed for time, this might assist you in resisting the urge to grab junk food or unhealthy snacks from a fast food restaurant. You may find it convenient to set aside some time on the weekends to prepare meals for the next week. You may make nutritious snacks and meals that are convenient to take on the move, such as cut vegetables, eggs that have been hard-boiled, or salads that have already been prepared. The following are some suggestions for meal preparation:

- Creating a food plan for the week in advance is highly recommended.
- Creating and adhering to a shopping list can help you avoid making impulsive purchases.
- Preparing a large amount of food at once in order to have leftovers for either lunch or supper the following day
- Making meal preparation simpler and more efficient by using helpful appliances in the kitchen, such as a slow cooker or pressure cooker.

Using healthy meal delivery services or meal kit delivery services, which include pre-measured materials and recipes for healthy meals, is yet another method to save time in the kitchen. These services may be found online. This might help you save time when it comes to going food shopping and preparing meals.

In a nutshell, keep in mind that it is perfectly OK to seek assistance. If you have a full agenda, you may want to think about asking family members for assistance with some responsibilities or hiring a professional to assist you with activities such as cleaning or looking after children. Because of this, you may have more time on your hands to devote to achieving your health and weight reduction objectives.

Plateaus

When you have been losing weight steadily, but all of a sudden your progress stops, and you are no longer seeing results, you have reached a weight loss plateau. This might be disheartening, but it's vital to recognize that weight loss plateaus are a normal part of the road to a healthier weight, and that virtually everyone experiences them at some point.

Altering your routine in some way is required in order for you to break through a weight loss rut that you have found yourself in. The following are some pointers that can assist you in navigating this difficult phase:

- *Change up your exercise routine:* Over time, your body will adapt to the same workout routine, and as a consequence, your rate of weight loss may slow or even stop. To get around this, consider working out more intensely or adding new exercises to your routine. Both of these strategies should help. For example, if you do a lot of cardiovascular exercise, you might want to add strength training to your normal routine.

- *Adjust your calorie intake:* Make adjustments to your calorie intake because, as you lose weight, your body will need fewer calories to operate normally, and the calorie deficit you are now experiencing may no longer be adequate for you to continue losing weight. If you want to get over this obstacle, consider cutting down on the number of calories you consume each day. But you should be careful not to cut your calorie intake by too much, because that could slow down your metabolism and make it harder for you to lose weight.

- *Focus on non-scale victories:* Weight reduction is not simply about the number that appears on the scale. Instead, you ought to concentrate on the victories that the scale does not account for. Other achievements, like being able to fit into smaller clothes or feeling more alive, should also be celebrated. This will help you remain motivated and serve as a reminder that you are making progress even if the scale is not moving.

- *Stay consistent*: Although reaching a plateau in your weight loss might be discouraging, it is essential to maintain your consistency with your healthy routines. Continue to eat a healthy diet, move your body often, and get enough sleep. Your body will start to adapt, and when it does, you'll find that your weight reduction continues.

Consider consulting with a professional: If you are having trouble breaking through a weight loss plateau, you may want to think about getting some expert advice from a personal trainer, a nutritionist, or a healthcare professional. They will be able to assist you in determining if there are any problems with your food or workout program, as well as provide direction for how to break through the plateau.

Keep in mind that shedding extra pounds is a process that takes time and requires you to be patient and consistent in your efforts. You can get past weight loss plateaus and keep making progress toward your goal if you have the right mindset and use the right strategies.

Temptations

While trying to lose weight, you will inevitably face temptations, and it might be difficult to stay strong in the face of such temptations. On the other hand, there are things you can do that might help you resist temptations and stay on track with your weight loss goals.

The ability to plan ahead is one of the keys to success in any approach. For instance, if you are aware that you will soon be attending a party or other social event at which unhealthy foods will be offered, you should make preparations in advance by either consuming a nutritious meal before attending the event or bringing your own nutritious snack from home. It is possible that doing this will prevent you from overindulging in meals that are rich in calories but lacking in nutrients.

Another technique is to make sure that you have access to healthy food selections at all times. It is important to stock your house with nutritious snacks, such as fruits, vegetables, and nuts, but you should steer clear of storing junk food there. When you are hungry, it will be easier for you to avoid giving in to the temptation of indulging in foods that are not good for you if you do this.

One more thing that might help is to get close friends and family members involved in what you are doing. If you have a friend or family member who is also attempting to reduce their weight or lead a healthier lifestyle, make a plan to exercise or cook nutritious meals together. This may give people incentive and a sense of responsibility, which will make it easier to avoid giving in to temptations.

Discovering the underlying causes of your temptations may be helpful in overcoming them. This should be done in addition to making plans ahead of time and keeping a variety of healthy options nearby. Do you suffer from stress, or do you just have nothing to do? Do you use food as a source of solace or as a means to numb or deal with bad emotions? If you deal with the problems that are causing your temptations, you will be able to develop better ways to deal with them and be less likely to give in to them.

Keep in mind that indulging in a guilty pleasure every once in a while is not only acceptable but encouraged. It is not only impossible, but also harmful, to entirely deny yourself all of the meals and activities that you like doing the most. Nonetheless, it is necessary to exercise self-control and strike a balance between competing priorities. Enjoy some of your favorite treats every now and then, but don't overdo it.

Instead, try to balance out the bad effects of these treats by making other, healthier choices throughout the day or week.

In general, if you want to reach your weight loss goals, you need to be consistent, patient, and committed. It can also be helpful to ask for help from friends, family, or a health care professional. Keep in mind that achieving long-term weight reduction is a process that calls for adjustments to lifestyle, not fast cures.

Conclusion

Final Thoughts and Actionable Steps for Achieving Fast and Healthy Weight Loss

The path to a healthier weight is one that is difficult and involves patience, self-control, and dedication. With the right attitude, tools, and support, it is possible to lose weight in a healthy way and keep it off. In this article, we talked about different ways to lose weight quickly and healthily, such as setting realistic goals, choosing healthy foods, working out regularly, dealing with stress, holding yourself accountable, and avoiding fad diets. In this last section, we'll summarize these strategies and show you how to put them into practice in your everyday life.

- *Set Realistic Goals*

One of the most important things you can do to achieve sustainable weight loss is to set realistic goals. Start by determining your current weight and ideal weight. From there, create a plan for losing weight at a rate of 1-2 pounds per week. This is a safe and realistic rate of weight loss that can be sustained over time.

In addition to weight loss goals, set achievable goals for exercising and eating healthy. For example, aim to exercise for 30 minutes a day or to eat five servings of fruits and vegetables each day. By setting achievable goals, you can build momentum and see progress, which can help you stay motivated.

- *Make Healthy Food Choices*

Eating a healthy, balanced diet is essential for sustainable weight loss. Make it a priority to consume a diet rich in fruits, vegetables, whole grains, lean proteins, and nutritious fats. These foods are nutrient-dense and low in calories, which can help you feel full and satisfied. Steer clear of processed meals that are rich in calories, as well as sugary beverages and snacks.

One helpful tip for making healthy food choices is to plan your meals in advance. This can help you avoid making decisions on the spot and make sure you have healthy choices available all day long. Another tip is to keep healthy snacks on hand, such as fresh fruit, nuts, or vegetables with hummus. By making healthy food choices, you can fuel your body with the nutrients it needs to support your weight loss goals.

- *Exercise Regularly*

Exercise is another important factor in sustainable weight loss. On most days of the week, strive to do physical activity lasting at least 30 minutes at a moderate intensity. You can do a variety of activities, such as walking, jogging, cycling, swimming, or dancing. Choose a pastime that you take pleasure in and make it a standard part of your daily routine.

One way to stay motivated to exercise is to set specific goals. For example, aim to run a 5K race or increase your strength and endurance. You may also keep tabs on your development and reward yourself for reaching milestones along the way. By exercising regularly, you can improve your overall health and well-being while supporting your weight loss goals.

- *Manage Stress*

Stress can have a negative impact on weight loss efforts. It can lead to emotional eating and make it harder to stick to healthy habits. Find ways to manage stress, such as meditation, yoga, deep breathing, or a relaxing hobby. Obtaining adequate sleep is another crucial component of an effective stress management strategy.

Another helpful tip for managing stress is to prioritize self-care. This can include taking time for yourself each day to do something you enjoy, such as reading a book, taking a bath, or listening to music. By managing stress, you can support your weight loss efforts and improve your overall well-being.

- *Stay Accountable*

Maintaining your weight reduction goals and staying on track might be easier if you have a support system.

Find a friend or family member who can encourage and motivate you. You can also join a weight loss group or work with a personal trainer or nutritionist to help you stay accountable.

Another helpful tip for staying accountable is to track your progress. This can include taking measurements, weighing yourself, or keeping a food journal. By tracking your progress, you can see how far you have come and where you still need to go to reach your goals. You can keep track of your progress in a number of ways, such as by measuring yourself, weighing yourself, or keeping a food diary. This will assist you in maintaining your motivation and keeping on track..

Another essential factor in achieving fast and healthy weight loss is getting enough sleep. The inability to get enough sleep may wreak havoc on your metabolism, making it more difficult to shed unwanted pounds.
Aim for 7-8 hours of sleep each night to support your weight loss efforts.

In addition to getting enough sleep, managing stress is also important. Emotional eating may be triggered by stress, which can be counterproductive to your attempts to lose weight. Discover healthy methods to deal with stress, such as meditation, taking slow, deep breaths, or engaging in an activity that you find pleasant.

It's also important to set realistic goals. Be honest with yourself about the amount of weight you can reduce and how soon it can happen. It's better to aim for a slow and steady weight loss of 1-2 pounds per week rather than trying to lose a lot of weight quickly. Also, set achievable goals such as exercising for 30 minutes a day, or reducing your calorie intake by a certain amount.

Making healthy food choices is essential for sustainable weight loss. Consume a diet rich in fresh fruits, vegetables, grains, lean proteins, and healthy fats. Steer clear of processed meals as well as high-calorie beverages and snacks. Eat meals that are low in calories but rich in nutrients if you want to be able to feel full and satisfied after eating.

Exercise is another important factor in sustainable weight loss. Try to do at least 30 minutes of moderate exercise on most days of the week.

You can do a variety of activities, such as walking, jogging, cycling, swimming, or dancing. Pick something that you take pleasure in doing, and make it a consistent part of your daily routine.

If you have people who will help you stay on track with your weight loss goals, it will be easier for you to lose weight. Find a friend or family member who can encourage and motivate you. You can also join a weight loss group or work with a personal trainer or nutritionist to help you stay accountable.

Avoid fad diets as they may promise quick weight loss, but they are not sustainable and can be harmful to your health. Avoid diets that force you to give up whole food groups or eat very few calories. Instead, focus on making healthy lifestyle changes that you can maintain in the long run.

With the right strategies, you can get past common problems like not being motivated, eating out of emotions, being too busy, hitting a plateau, and giving in to temptations. For example, find ways to stay motivated, such as by reminding yourself of the reasons why you started your weight loss journey or seeking inspiration from success stories. Find healthy ways to deal with stress or keep a food journal to figure out what makes you eat out of emotion.

If you have a busy schedule, put your health first by planning time to exercise and make meals. To get past a plateau, try switching up your workout routine, making your workouts harder, or changing how many calories you eat.

Finally, for temptations, make a plan for dealing with them, such as having healthy snacks on hand or scheduling workouts with a friend.

In conclusion, to lose weight quickly and healthily, you need to do a number of things, such as make healthy food choices, exercise regularly, deal with stress, get enough sleep, track your progress, have a support system, and stay away from fad diets.

It's important to be patient, consistent, and flexible in your approach, as weight loss is a journey that requires time and effort. You can reach your weight loss goals and live a healthier, happier life by making changes to your lifestyle that you can keep up with.

Julie K. Geneva